Monoclonal Antibodies to Neural Antigens

REPORT OF A MEETING SUPPORTED BY
The Marie H. Robertson Fund for Neurobiology

Cold Spring Harbor Reports in the Neurosciences • Volume 2

Monoclonal Antibodies to Neural Antigens

Edited by

RONALD McKAY
Cold Spring Harbor Laboratory

MARTIN C. RAFF
University College London

LOUIS F. REICHARDT
University of California, San Francisco

Cold Spring Harbor Laboratory
1981

Cold Spring Harbor Reports in the Neurosciences

Volume 1 • Molluscan Nerve Cells: From Biophysics to Behavior
Volume 2 • Monoclonal Antibodies to Neural Antigens

Monoclonal Antibodies to Neural Antigens
©1981 by Cold Spring Harbor Laboratory
All rights reserved
Printed in the United States of America
Cover and book designed by Emily Harste

Library of Congress Cataloging in Publication Data
Main entry under title:

Monoclonal antibodies to neural antigens.

(Cold Spring Harbor reports in the neurosciences, ISSN 0276-4695 ; v. 2)
Report of a meeting held at Banbury Center
of Cold Spring Harbor Laboratory, Nov. 5–8,
1980.
Includes index.
1. Nervous system—Congresses. 2. Tissue
specific antibodies—Congresses. 3. Gammo-
pathies, Monoclonal—Congresses. 4. Immuno-
specificity—Congresses. I. McKay, Ronald
D. G. II. Raff, Martin C. III. Reichardt,
Louis F. IV. Series. [DNLM: 1. Antibodies.
2. Antigens. 3. Antigen-antibody reactions.
4. Clone cells. 5. Nervous system—Physiology.
W1 C0133E v. 2 / WL 102 M754]
QP361.M819   599.01'88   81-10185
ISBN 0-87969-138-7   AACR2

All Cold Spring Harbor Laboratory publications are available through booksellers or
may be ordered directly from Cold Spring Harbor Laboratory, Box 100, Cold Spring
Harbor, New York 11724.

Participants

Richard Akeson
Department of Cell Biology
Children's Hospital Research Foundation
Cincinnati, Ohio 45229

Colin Barnstable
Department of Neurobiology
Harvard Medical School
Boston, Massachusetts 02115

Ellen K. Bayne
Department of Embryology
Carnegie Institution of Washington
Baltimore, Maryland 21210

Yoheved Berwald-Netter
Collège de France
Paris, France 75231

Steven Burden
Department of Anatomy
Harvard Medical School
Boston, Massachusetts 02115

Steven S. Carlson
Department of Biochemistry
University of California Medical Center
San Francisco, California 94143

Gary Ciment
Department of Biology
University of Oregon
Eugene, Oregon 97403

James Cohen
Department of Zoology
University College London
London, England WC1E 6BT

A. Claudio Cuello
Department of Pharmacology
University of Oxford
Oxford, England OX1 3QT

Angel DeBlas
Laboratory of Biochemical Genetics
National Heart, Lung, and Blood Institute
Bethesda, Maryland 20205

George Eisenbarth
Duke University Medical Center
Durham, North Carolina 27710

Kay Fields
Department of Neurology
Albert Einstein College of Medicine
Bronx, New York 10461

Sara Fuchs
Department of Chemical Immunology
The Weizmann Institute of Science
Rehovot, Israel

Gregory Giotta
Department of Developmental Biology
Salk Institute
San Diego, California 92138

David Gottlieb
Department of Anatomy and Neurobiology
Washington University School of Medicine
St. Louis, Missouri 63110

Stephen Heinemann
Department of Neurobiology
Salk Institute
San Diego, California 92138

Harvey J. Karten
Department of Psychiatry and Behavioral Sciences
State University of New York
Stony Brook, New York 11794

Regis Kelly
Department of Biochemistry
University of California
San Francisco, California 94143

Lois A. Lampson
Department of Anatomy
University of Pennsylvania School of Medicine
Philadelphia, Pennsylvania 19104

Gregory Lemke
Department of Biology
California Institute of Technology
Pasadena, California 91125

William Matthew
Department of Biochemistry
University of California
San Francisco, California 94143

Marshall Nirenberg
Laboratory of Biochemical Genetics
National Heart, Lung, and Blood Institute
Bethesda, Maryland 20205

Ronald McKay
Cold Spring Harbor Laboratory
Cold Spring Harbor, New York 11724

Rebecca Pruss
Laboratory of Clinical Science
National Institute of Arthritis, Metabolism, and Digestive Diseases
Bethesda, Maryland 20205

Martin C. Raff
Department of Zoology
University College London
London, England WC1E 6BT

Louis F. Reichardt
Department of Physiology
University of California
San Francisco, California 94143

Elizabeth Ross
Department of Neurobiology
Cornell University Medical College
New York, New York 10021

Melitta Schachner
Department of Neurobiology
University of Heidelberg
Heidelberg, Federal Republic of Germany D6900

Michael D. Schneider
Laboratory of Biochemical Genetics
National Heart, Lung, and Blood Institute
Bethesda, Maryland 20205

William Stallcup
Salk Institute
San Diego, California 92138

Charles F. Stevens
Department of Physiology
Yale School of Medicine
New Haven, Connecticut 06510

G. David Trisler
Laboratory of Biochemical Genetics
National Heart, Lung, and Blood Institute
Bethesda, Maryland 20205

Birgit Zipser
Cold Spring Harbor Laboratory
Cold Spring Harbor, New York 11724

Transcribing Editors

Richard Chaillet
Department of Physiology
Yale University School of Medicine
New Haven, Connecticut 06510

Shinobu C. Fujita
Division of Biology
California Institute of Technology
Pasadena, California 91125

Michael D. Schneider
Laboratory of Biochemical Genetics
National Heart, Lung, and Blood Institute
Bethesda, Maryland 20205

Janet Winter
Department of Zoology
University College London
London, England WC1E 6BT

Eve Wolinsky
Department of Neurobiology
Harvard Medical School
Boston, Massachusetts 02115

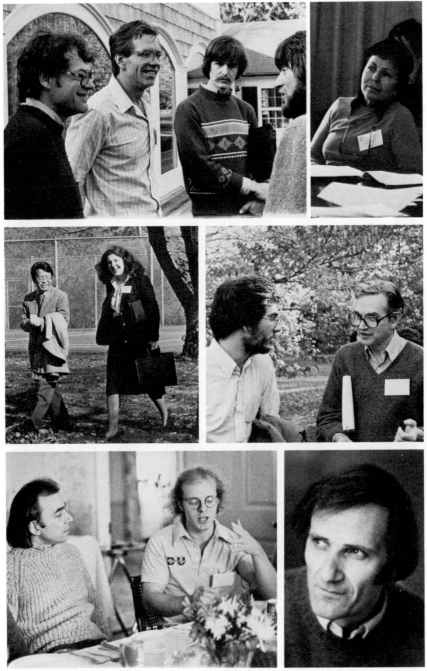

First row: C.F. Stevens, L.F. Reichardt, C. Barnstable, R. Kelly; S. Fuchs
Second row: T.H. Joh, E. Ross; R. Chaillet, M. Nirenberg
Third row: R. McKay, G. Lemke; M.C. Raff

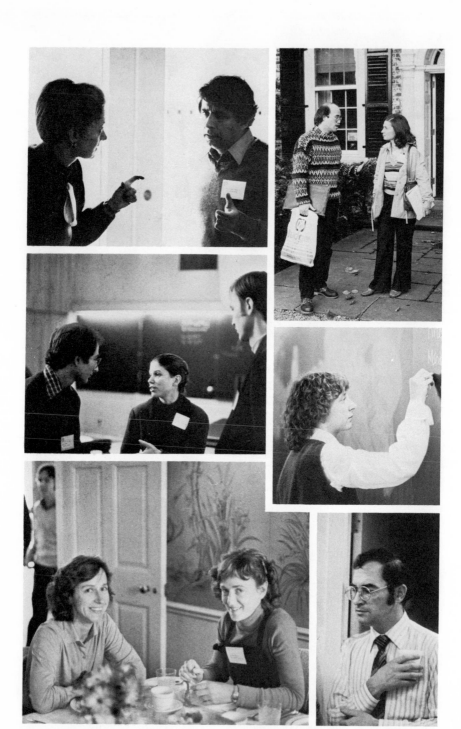

First row: M. Schachner, A.C. Cuello; S. Burden, E. Bayne
Second row: G. Ciment, K. Fields, R. Akeson; R.M. Pruss
Third row: B. Zipser, S. Hockfield; H. Karten

Preface

This volume presents summaries of talks given at a meeting held at the Banbury Conference Center of Cold Spring Harbor Laboratory in the autumn of 1980. The meeting was intended to be an informal workshop for scientists engaged in exploring the application of hybridoma technology to the nervous system. Their contributions were painstakingly transcribed and shaped into chapters by a group of "scribes" (Richard Chaillet, Shinobu Fujita, Michael Schneider, Janet Winter, and Eve Wolinsky) who attended the conference, and then each chapter was edited by the authors and the book editors. By this process we hoped to produce a book that would make this field generally accessible and would help to define the questions in neurobiology that may be answered using this new technique.

There are at least four requirements for a good meeting: (1) an exciting intellectual problem that is experimentally accessible; (2) the experimenters; (3) a pleasant meeting place; and (4) the funds that allow us to travel and talk. In focusing on the use of monoclonal antibodies as probes in neurobiology, a technology with great potential and an increasing list of achievements, we were assured of lively discussion. The participants, all directly involved in applying this technique, were able to gather in the relaxed environment of the Banbury Conference Center, with funds for this exchange of ideas being generously provided by the Marie H. Robertson Fund for Neurobiology. Encouraged by the success of the meeting, we now hope that the resulting book will contribute to the development of this field.

For assisting us in achieving these goals, we owe thanks first of all to those in the Laboratory's meetings office, especially Gladys Kist, who helped organize the meeting. Thanks also go to the Publications Department of Cold Spring Harbor, in particular to our technical editor, Douglas Owen. They all remained cheerful when we broke our schedules and failed to provide manuscripts on time.

Sponsoring a meeting on a subject with few publications requires a commitment to new research and an appreciation of what is possible. We hope that the forthcoming work in this field justifies Jim Watson's enthusiastic support, which made both the meeting and this book possible.

Ronald McKay
Martin C. Raff
Louis F. Reichardt

Contents

V.   The Neuromuscular Junction

Monoclonal Antibodies to Neural Antigens

Introduction

RONALD McKAY, MARTIN C. RAFF, and LOUIS F. REICHARDT

I. IMMUNOLOGY AND NEUROBIOLOGY

• Our knowledge of the nervous system has been dramatically improved through the use of antisera obtained by conventional procedures from the blood of immunized animals. Some sera distinguish among a variety of neuronal and nonneuronal cell types. Antisera to antigens of the major cell classes in the central and peripheral nervous systems have been used to identify, purify, or destroy these cells in vitro (see, e.g., Raff et al. 1979). Some of these antisera, specific for cell classes, are proving invaluable in identifying cell lineages and factors necessary for normal cellular proliferation and differentiation (see, e.g., Brockes et al. 1980).

Neurobiologists have also used antisera to identify and characterize the components of electrical and chemical synapses, which are the sites of cell-to-cell communication in the nervous system. Antisera to purified calmodulin, clathrin, and tubulin have demonstrated their specific localization to synaptic regions (Matus et al. 1975; Cheng et al. 1980; Wood et al. 1980), generating hypotheses on the function in the synapse of these localized concentrations of molecules that are essential for the normal function of virtually every cell type. Antisera have been made that reveal the presence at the neuromuscular junction of antigens specific to the synaptic region of the basal lamina (Sanes and Hall 1979); this region plays an important role in the formation and function of this synapse. These antisera are potentially powerful probes for identifying the factors in this specialized region that have been shown to induce differentiation of nerve and muscle (Sanes et al. 1978; Burden et al. 1979).

1

Many factors that appear to regulate the expression of differentiated functions in classes of neurons have been reported, and immunological studies have been critical in establishing their biological roles. For example, the biological importance of nerve growth factor (NGF) was established by injection of anti-NGF antibodies into neonatal mice. These injections induced virtually complete destruction of the sympathetic nervous system (Levi-Montalcini and Booker 1960). Other factors essential for survival, proliferation, transmitter choice, neurite growth, or steps in synaptogenesis of neurons grown in culture have recently been described (Patterson and Chun 1977; Collins 1978; Adler et al. 1979, 1981; Ebendahl et al. 1979; Jessel et al. 1979; Nishi and Berg 1979; Collins and Garrett 1980; Coughlin et al. 1981). In each case, the use of antibodies will likely be critical in demonstrating biological relevance.

Finally, great progress has resulted from the use of antibodies to neuropeptides, transmitter biosynthetic enzymes, and nonpeptide transmitters in order to identify the cells in different parts of the nervous system that contain these molecules and are therefore likely to use them as transmitters. More than 20 transmitter candidates have been localized to neuronal classes by means of immunocytochemical procedures (Snyder and Innis 1979; Stell et al. 1980). Such studies have provided the anatomical basis for a more-detailed understanding of neuronal circuitry and have stimulated electrophysiological experiments to test the functions of these transmitter candidates (see, e.g., Morita et al. 1980; Nicoll et al. 1980).

Although conventionally prepared antibodies have made an important contribution to our current understanding of the nervous system, it has been clear for many years that their utility is limited by shortcomings difficult to surmount when using neural preparations. Even when a highly purified molecule is used as the immunogen, these antisera almost always contain antibody molecules that recognize different antigenic determinants and have different affinities. Furthermore, it is often not possible to obtain such a purified molecule from the nervous system; such compounds may be present only in very low quantities. Even the isolation of pure populations of cells or organelles has often been beyond the power of the methods available (see, e.g., Matus and Taff-Jones 1978; Kelly et al. 1979). Neurobiologists are not even certain which molecules should be purified in some situations (e.g., attempts to purify cell-surface molecules thought to be specific for neuronal classes or developmental stages). Yet immunization with impure preparations is problematic: Even though the antiserum may contain antibodies to the cell or organelle of interest, its efficiency will most likely be compromised by the presence of antibodies to other molecules. Clearly, methods to obtain specific antisera by using heterogeneous immunogens would be particularly valuable in studies of the nervous system.

An important element in our current understanding of the immune response is that a single immunoglobulin (Ig)-secreting cell and its progeny synthesize only a single type of antibody. Thus, the antigen-combining sites in the immunoglobulin secreted by a cell will have a single amino acid sequence and specificity for binding antigen that is comparable to that of enzymes for their substrates (Burnet 1957). This feature of the immune system suggested a possible means to reduce the complexity of a standard antiserum. If clones of single Ig-secreting cells could be propagated in culture, monospecific (or monoclonal) antibodies could be obtained from immunizations with heterogeneous or polyspecific antigens. Monoclonal antibodies could be generated that distinguish among closely related neuropeptides and their precursors by their primary amino acid sequences. The different functional domains of receptors or enzymes could be recognized by monospecific antibodies. In all cases, such antibodies would be produced without contamination by antibodies to antigens other than those of interest.

Ig-secreting cells were first adapted to continuous culture by fusing them with a transformed cell line of the immune system (Köhler and Milstein 1975). These hybrid cells, termed hybridomas, combine continuous viability in cell culture with the ability to produce antibody molecules that have only one antigen-binding specificity. Appropriate selection procedures allow the investigator to identify and isolate those cells producing antibodies of interest from the mixture of Ig-secreting hybrid cells generated in a fusion. In the last six years, similar cell lines have been isolated that secrete monoclonal antibodies to a wide variety of antigens that are of particular interest to neurobiologists; these include neuropeptides, transmitter biosynthetic enzymes, cytoskeletal elements, receptors, synaptic vesicles, and cell-surface markers. These antibodies have revealed a large number of antigenic differences among neuronal classes. We now anticipate that such antigenic distinctions will eventually divide neurons into at least as many classes as have been described on morphological grounds by Cajal and other neuroanatomists. In the future, monoclonal antibodies will undoubtedly be widely used by neurobiologists in classical neuroanatomical studies as reagents to purify defined cell types in vitro or ablate them in vivo and to identify factors required for normal development or synaptogenesis.

II. NOTES ON ANTIBODIES AND HYBRIDOMA TECHNOLOGY

• To understand the papers in this collection, one must be familiar with some basic properties of the immune system. The following section is designed as an introduction to some of the concepts and the literature relevant to generating antibody-secreting cell lines and characterizing the specificity of their monoclonal antibodies. Immunoglobulins, which are present in the circulation of all vertebrates, have the unusual property of binding tightly to a wide range of different molecules. The structure of immunoglobulins and the exquisite genetic basis of antibody diversity are now well understood.

Specificity

The nature of the antibody-combining site and the affinity of antigen-antibody interactions have been extensively studied. The affinity constant, K_a, ranges widely from 10^5 to 10^9 M^{-1} (Karush 1962). The specificity of antibody-antigen interaction, however, is not absolute, and it has been argued that antibodies have evolved to bind more than one antigen (Richards 1975). Consequently, antigenic cross-reactivity is not equivalent to molecular identity; cross-reactivity only indicates that two molecules share some antigenic determinants. However, since even a single amino acid change within a determinant can lead to enormous differences in antibody binding (Clevinger 1980), it has been possible to produce antisera that discriminate between chemically similar antigens, e.g., leucine and methionine enkephalins.

Complexity of Antisera

Estimates of the number of different antigen-binding sites possible among the antibodies that a mouse can generate vary, but this number is larger than 10^7 (Klinman and Press 1975; Köhler and Milstein 1976; Sigal and Klinman 1978; Cancro et al. 1979; Hood 1981; Leder 1981; Tonegawa 1981). This great diversity is almost certainly essential to protect warm-blooded animals from a plethora of pathogens, some of which have evolved sophisticated mechanisms to escape immune surveillance. As a consequence of this diversity, most antigens induce a very complex immune response — the production of antibodies containing different sequences that can bind different sites on each antigen. Heterogeneity of antiserum composition is a major technical problem in using antisera as scientific tools. Furthermore, this problem is compounded by the fact that the precise mixture of antibodies produced against a given antigen will vary from one animal to another and, with time, in a single immunized animal.

The immune response is modulated by selective expansion and differentiation of different populations of Ig-secreting cells. Single lymphocytes could not be responsive to specific antigens if they secreted antibodies with many different binding specificities. In fact, Burnet (1957) proposed that all the antibodies secreted by a single lymphocyte possess the same antigen-binding site. Direct measurements of the specificity of the antibodies secreted by single lymphocytes growing in microdrops have supported this concept (Nossal and

Lederberg 1958), which has been confirmed by studies demonstrating that the antibody molecules secreted by clonally derived, transformed, Ig-secreting cell lines have a unique amino acid sequence (Edelman 1973). Recently, a series of elegant studies on the structure of Ig genes has revealed many of the mechanisms that underlie this specificity (Seidman et al. 1978; Davis et al. 1980).

Antibody-secreting cells can be identified easily, but these cells can be maintained in culture for only short times (Klinman et al. 1977). Tumor derivatives of the immune system exist, and these cells have been very useful tools for studying, in isolation, the cellular components of the immune system. The myelomas are tumor cell lines that produce immunoglobulins. Induced myelomas have been used to study many features of immunoglobulin structure and synthesis and, more recently, to analyze the genetic basis of antibody diversity. These cell lines can be grown in continuous suspension culture, cloned, and genetically manipulated to yield variant immunoglobulins and drug-resistant cell lines (Cotton and Milstein 1973; Adetugbo et al. 1977; Margulies et al. 1977; Milstein et al. 1977). These studies, and the techniques of somatic cell genetics, provided the technical basis for the production of monoclonal antibodies to defined antigens.

Hybridoma Technology

Köhler and Milstein (1975, 1976) were the first to devise a procedure for generating hybridoma lines secreting antibodies to a chosen antigen. They used Sendai virus to fuse antibody-producing cells from the spleens of mice immunized with sheep red blood cells (SRBC) to a myeloma that lacked a purine salvage pathway enzyme (hypoxanthine phosphoribosyl transferase [HPRT]). The unfused spleen cells died because they were incapable of survival or proliferation in culture. The unfused myeloma cells were killed by inclusion of the drug aminopterin, which prevents de novo synthesis of purines. The only viable cell lines, called hybridomas, contained a functional HPRT gene from the spleen cells, allowing them to convert hypoxanthine into the essential purine nucleotides, and genes from the parent myeloma that enabled them to grow indefinitely in culture. This selection against the parent myeloma was essential since a very low frequency of viable hybridoma cells (10^{-4} to 10^{-5}) was generated in their procedure. Those cell lines secreting anti-SRBC antibodies were identified in a plaque assay. Surprisingly, the hybrid population contained a much greater frequency of anti-SRBC secreting clones than the lymphocyte population in the original spleen ($\sim$ 10% vs 0.01%), implying that antigen-stimulated cells have a high probability of yielding viable hybrids.

Similar procedures, usually using polyethylene glycol instead of Sendai virus to fuse cells, have demonstrated that hybrid cells that secrete antibodies to many different types of antigens can be isolated (see this volume). There are a large number of parameters that influence the success of obtaining particular antibodies, the most important of which is the immune response of the immunized animal (Lake et al. 1979; Fazekas de St. Groth and Scheidegger 1980). The frequency of hybrids obtained from different fusions reflects the percentage of B lymphocytes in the spleen directed against that antigen, so it is important to induce an effective immune response (Lake et al. 1979). For example, one cannot expect to obtain hybrids if the animal is tolerant to the antigen and lacking reactive lymphocytes in its spleen.

Table 1
Myeloma Cell Lines

Cell line	Ig synthesized	Species	Reference
X63-Ag8	γ, κ	mouse	1
NS1-Ag4/1	κ	mouse	2
X63-Ag8.6.5.3	none	mouse	3
SP2/0-Ag14	none	mouse	4
FO	none	mouse	5
S194/5XX0.BU.1	none	mouse	6
MPC11-45.6TG1	γ_{2b}, κ	mouse	7
210.RCY3.Ag1.2.3	κ	rat	8,9
U-266AR$_1$	λ	man	10,11

Many of these myeloma lines and hybrids derived from them are available from the Cell Distribution Center, The Salk Institute, P.O. Box 1809, San Diego, California 92112. Tel. 714-453-4100; TWX 910 337 1283 SALK LILA.
Original papers on hybridoma technology:
1. Köhler, G. and C. Milstein. 1975. *Nature* **256**:495.
2. Köhler, G. and C. Milstein. 1976. *Eur. J. Immunol.* **6**:511.
3. Kearney, J.F., A. Radbruch, B. Liesegang, and K. Rajewsky. 1979. *J. Immunol.* **123**:1548.
4. Shulman, M., C.D. Wilde, and G. Köhler. 1978. *Nature* **276**:269.
5. Fazekas de St. Groth, S. and D. Scheidegger. 1980. *J. Immunol. Methods* **34**:1.
6. Trowbridge, I.S. 1978. Interspecies spleen-myeloma hybrid producing monoclonal antibody against mouse lymphocyte surface glycoprotein, T200. *J. Exp. Med.* **148**:313.
7. Margulies, D.H., W.M. Kuehl, and M.D. Scharff. 1976. *Cell* **8**:405.
8. Gefter, M.L., D.H. Margulies, and M.D. Scharff. 1977. *Somat. Cell Genet.* **3**:213.
9. Galfre, G., C. Milstein, and B. Wright. 1979. *Nature* **277**:131.
10. Marshak-Rothstein, A., P. Fink, T. Gridley, D.H. Raulet, M.J. Beran, and M.L. Gefter. 1979. *J. Immunol.* **122**:2491.
11. Olsson, L. and H.S. Kaplan. 1980. *Proc. Natl. Acad. Sci.* **77**:5429.
12. Galfre, G., S.C. Howe, C. Milstein, G.W. Butcher, and J.C. Howard. 1977. *Nature* **266**:550.
13. Köhler, G., T. Pearson, and C. Milstein. 1977. *Somat. Cell Genet.* **3**:303.
14. Köhler, G. 1976. *Eur. J. Immunol.* **6**:340.

The time between the final immunization and the harvesting of cells from the spleen is critical, and the optimum time varies for different antigens (Lake et al. 1979). Furthermore, a number of different myeloma parent cell lines (listed in Table 1) that differ in their fusion efficiency and other properties are available. Also, several modifications of the fusion procedure that affect the efficiency of fusion and may affect the probability of obtaining certain types of clones have been reported (Fazekas de St. Groth and Scheidegger 1980).

Although the vast majority of the currently available hybridoma cell lines have been generated using the methods described above, a number of other procedures are being developed and may be more widely used in the future. First, procedures for challenging cultured spleen cells with antigen in vitro and then fusing these cultured cells have been reported. These procedures appear to require very small quantities of antigen (Lubin and Mohler 1980). Second, several viruses have been used to transform immunoglobulin-secreting cells directly. For example, Epstein-Barr virus transformation of human lymphocytes has yielded cell lines secreting antibodies specific for several antigens, diphtheria (Tsuchiya et al. 1980) and tetanus toxin (Zurawski 1978). Even though current viral transformation procedures are not efficient enough for general use, technical developments in this field may make direct transformation more attractive in the future. In addition, recent successes in developing growth-factor-supplemented culture systems that permit the long-term proliferation of untransformed T lymphocytes suggest that the continuous propagation of B-lymphocyte clones will soon be possible (Nabel et al. 1981).

Several more-detailed reviews of hybridoma technology are available (Potter and Melchers 1978; Melchers et al. 1979; Kennett et al. 1980; Mishell and Shugi 1980; van Vunakis and Langone 1980; Fellows and Eisenbarth 1981).

Detection and Characterization of Antibodies

This volume presents discussions of monoclonal antibodies that identify many different types of molecules with different roles in the nervous system. These include antibodies to transmitters, neuropeptides, receptors, enzymes, and subcellular structures such as synaptic vesicles. In addition, antibodies are reported that distinguish cell types in the nervous system. In the many experimental reports, different approaches have been used to obtain antibodies of interest. The two features of experimental design that determine the outcome are the choice of antigen and the procedure for screening hybrid clones. Several groups have sought antibodies to a particular molecule and have used purified, well-characterized antigens to immunize mice. At the other extreme, antibodies have been raised against a whole invertebrate nervous system or portions of the mammalian nervous system. In these cases, thousands of different molecules are injected into a mouse.

Solid-phase radioimmunoassays provide sensitive probes for antibodies that bind purified antigens (Klinman 1972; O'Sullivan et al. 1979). With a complex antiserum to a mixture of antigens, a solid-phase assay does not immediately identify the subset of antibodies of interest, but with monoclonal antibodies, identification is straightforward. This facilitates the cloning of antibody-secreting hybridoma cell lines. When fractions of tissues or cells, rather than purified antigens, are used in solid-phase assays, monoclonal antibodies can be shown to bind antigens that have been enriched in particular cell types or tissue fractions. However, these complex comparisons are subject to a variety of artifacts. If a sufficiently precise screening procedure is available, monoclonal antibodies to particular molecules can be obtained using a heterogeneous immunogen; e.g., monoclonal antibodies to the human histocompatibility antigens (Barnstable et al. 1978; Hammerling et al. 1978) and interferon (Secher and Burke 1980) have been obtained in this way. Contributions to this book indicate that these procedures will be widely used by neurobiologists to make specific antibodies to molecules that are very difficult to purify to homogeneity.

Uses of Monoclonal Antibodies

The use of monoclonal antibodies to *identify* molecules of interest is straightforward. Many molecules that are now well studied were first identified with antibodies. Antibodies may also be used to *purify* antigens of interest. Although this approach was initially technically difficult, the histocompatibility antigens, the acetylcholine receptor, and interferon have all now been purified using immunoaffinity chromatography (Hermann and Mescher 1979; Parham 1979; Lennon et al. 1980; Secher and Burke 1980).

A range of monoclonal antibodies may then be used to analyze in detail the *structure and functions* of an antigen. The histocompatibility antigens and the tumor antigen of the SV40 virus are the best-studied examples. In both cases, a number of monoclonal antibodies that bind to different antigenic sites on these molecules are known.

Antibodies can be used to study the *differentiation and ontogeny of cells*. In the cells of the immune system, two types of tissue distribution have been reported. Many antigens, termed lineage antigens, are expressed on cells in a manner that is consistent with our knowledge of the differentiation of those cells. For example, the common leukocyte antigen (CLA) appears to recognize all cells of leukocyte origin (for review, see Springer 1980). In contrast, other antigens, such as heat-stable antigen (HSA) and Thy-1, are present on many cell types that are not of the same lineage (Marshak-Rothstein et al. 1979; Springer 1980). The underlying basis for the irregular expression of this class of antigens, termed jumping antigens, is not yet clear, but it appears that single antigenic markers cannot be used alone as proof of an ontogenic relationship between cells in the nervous system.

Antibodies also allow the *purification of cells*. The power of this approach was first demonstrated by separation and reconstitution of the different cell types of the immune system. During the past several years, Raff and his colleagues (Raff et al. 1979) have attempted to identify antigenic markers for the major cell types in the nervous system, with the aim of developing procedures for purifying and culturing defined neural cell types and studying their interactions. They have now defined cell-surface markers that distinguish the major types of cell in the nervous system. These procedures have already greatly contributed to studies on Schwann-cell proliferation and differentiation. Presentations at the meeting made it evident that antibodies will be powerful reagents for separating and studying the many known classes of cells in the nervous system.

Antibodies can be used to study the *function of specific molecules or cells in the nervous system*. Antisera to NGF, for example, specifically destroy sympathetic and sensory neurons in vivo (Johnson et al. 1980). Antibodies to other factors can be expected to destroy other neuronal populations, identifying the cells that require these substances. Recently, it has become possible to destroy cells more directly by incubation with specific antibodies coupled to cytotoxic agents. Ultimately, therefore, we may be able to study the behavioral consequences in the whole animal of removing precisely defined groups of cells in the nervous system with monoclonal antibodies.

REFERENCES

Adetugbo, K., C. Milstein, and D.S. Secher. 1977. Molecular analysis of spontaneous somatic mutants. *Nature* **265**:299.

Adler, R. and S. Varon. 1981. Neuritic guidance by polyornithine-attached materials of ganglionic origin. *Dev. Biol.* **81**:1.

Adler, R., K.B. Landa, M. Manthorpe, and S. Varon. 1979. Cholinergic neuronotrophic factors. V. Segregation of survival- and neurite-promoting activities in heart-conditioned media. *Brain Res.* **188**:437.

Barnstable, C.J., W. F. Bodmer, G. Brown, G. Galfre, C. Milstein, A.F. Williams, and A. Ziegler. 1978. Production of monoclonal antibodies to group A erythrocytes, HLA and other human cell surface antigens— New tools for genetic analysis. *Cell* **14**:9.

Brockes, J.P., G.E. Lemke, and D.R. Balzer, Jr. 1980. Purification and preliminary characterization of a glial growth factor from the bovine pituitary. *J. Biol. Chem.* **255**:8374.

Burden, S.J., P.B. Sargent, and U.J. McMahan. 1979. Acetylcholine receptors in regenerating muscle accumulate at original synaptic sites in the absence of nerve. *J. Cell Biol.* **82:**412.

Burnet, F. 1957. A modification of Jerne's theory of antibody production using the concept of clonal selection. *Aust. J. Sci.* **20:**67.

Cancro, M.P., D.E. Wylie, W. Gerhard, and N.R. Klinman. 1979. Patterned acquisition of the antibody repertoire: Diversity of the hemagglutinin-specific B-cell repertoire in neonatal BALB/c mice. *Proc. Natl. Acad. Sci.* **76:**6577.

Cheng, T.P.-O., F.I. Byrd, J.N. Whittaker, and J.G. Wood. 1980. Immunocyto-chemical localization of coated vesicle protein in rodent nervous system. *J. Cell Biol.* **86:**624.

Clevinger, B., J. Schilling, L. Hood, and J.M. Davie. 1980. Structural correlates of cross-reactive and individual idiotypic determinants on murine antibodies to α-(1→3) dextran. *J. Exp. Med.* **151:**1059.

Collins, F. 1978. Axon initiation by ciliary neurons in culture. *Dev. Biol.* **65:**50.

Collins, F. and J.E. Garrett, Jr. 1980. Elongating nerve fibers are guided by a pathway of material released from embryonic non-neural cells. *Proc. Natl. Acad. Sci.* **77:**6226.

Cotton, R.G.H. and C. Milstein. 1973. Fusion of two immunoglobulin-producing myeloma cells. *Nature* **244:**42.

Coughlin, M.D., E.M. Bloom, and I.B. Black. 1981. Characterization of a neuronal growth factor from mouse heart-cell-conditioned medium. *Dev. Biol.* **82:**56.

Davis, M.M., S.K. Kim, and L. Hood. 1980. Immunoglobulin class switching: Developmentally regulated DNA rearrangements during differentiation. *Cell* **22:**1.

Ebendahl, T., M. Beleu, C.-O. Jacobson, and J. Porath. 1979. Neurite outgrowth elicited by embryonic chick heart: Partial purification of the active factor. *Neurosci. Lett.* **14:**91.

Edelman, G. 1973. Antibody structure and molecular immunology. *Science* **180:**830.

Fazekas de St. Groth, S. and D. Scheidegger. 1980. Production of monoclonal antibodies: Strategy and tactics. *J. Immunol. Methods* **35:**1.

Fellows, R.E. and G. Eisenbarth, eds. 1981. *Monoclonal antibodies in endocrine research.* Raven Press, New York. (In press.)

Hammerling, G.J., H. Lemke, U. Hammerling, C. Hohmann, R. Wallich, and K. Rajewsky. 1978. Monoclonal antibodies against murine cell surface antigens: Anti-H-2, anti-Id and anti-T cell antibodies. *Curr. Top. Microbiol. Immunol.* **81:**100.

Herrmann, S.H., and M.F. Mescher. 1979. Purification of the H-2K^k molecule of the murine major histocompatibility complex. *J. Biol. Chem.* **254:**8713.

Hood, L., M. Davis, P. Early, K. Calame, S. Kim, S. Crews, and H. Huang. 1981. Two types of DNA rearrangements in immunoglobulin genes. *Cold Spring Harbor Symp. Quant. Biol.* **45:**887.

Jessel, T.M., R.E. Siegel, and G.D. Fischbach. 1979. Induction of ACh receptors on cultured muscle by a factor extracted from brain and spinal cord. *Proc. Natl. Acad. Sci.* **76:**5397.

Johnson, E.M., P.D. Gorin, L.D. Brandeis, and J. Pearson. 1980. Dorsal root ganglion neurons are destroyed by exposure in utero to maternal antibody to nerve growth factor. *Science* **210**:916.

Karush, F. 1962. Immunological specificity and molecular structure. *Adv. Immunol.* **2**:1.

Kelly, R.B., J.W. Deutsch, S.S. Carlson, and J.A. Wagner. 1979. Biochemistry of neurotransmitter release. *Annu. Rev. Neurosci.* **2**:399.

Kennet, R.H., T.J. McKearn, and K.B. Bechtol, eds. 1980. *Monoclonal antibodies.* Plenum Press, New York.

Klinman, N.R. 1972. The mechanism of antigenic stimulation of primary and secondary clonal precursor cells. *J. Exp. Med.* **136**:241.

Klinman, N.R. and J.L. Press. 1975. The B cell specificity repertoire: Its relationship to definable subpopulations. *Transplant. Rev.* **24**:41.

Klinman, N., N. Sigal, E. Metcalf, S. Pierce, and P. Gearhart. 1977. The interplay of evolution and environment in B-cell diversification. *Cold Spring Harbor Symp. Quant. Biol.* **41**:165.

Köhler, G. and C. Milstein. 1975. Continuous cultures of fused cells secreting antibodies of predefined specificity. *Nature* **256**:495.

————. 1976. Derivation of specific antibody-producing tissue culture and tumor lines by cell fusion. *Eur. J. Immunol.* **6**:511.

Lake, P., E.A. Clarke, M. Khorshidi, and G.H. Sunshine. 1979. Production and characterization of cytotoxic Thy-1 antibody-secreting hybrid cell lines. Detection of T cell subsets. *Eur. J. Immunol.* **9**:875.

Leder, P., E.E. Max, J.G. Seidman, S.-P. Kwan, M. Scharff, M. Nau, and B. Norman. 1981. Recombination events that activate, diversify, and delete immunoglobulin genes. *Cold Spring Harbor Symp. Quant. Biol.* **45**:859.

Lennon, V.A., M. Thomson, and J. Chen. 1980. Properties of nicotinic acetylcholine receptors isolated by affinity chromatography on monoclonal antibodies. *J. Biol. Chem.* **255**:4395.

Levi-Montalcini, R. and B. Booker. 1960. Destruction of the sympathetic ganglia in mammals by an antiserum to NGF. *Proc. Natl. Acad. Sci.* **46**:384.

Lubin, R.A. and M.A. Mohler. 1980. *In vitro* immunization as an adjunct to the production of hybridomas producing antibodies against the lymphokine osteoclast activating factor. *Mol. Immunol.* **17**:635.

Margulies, D.H., W. Cieplinski, B. Dharmgrongartama, M.L. Gefter, S.L. Morrison, T. Kelly, and M.D. Scharff. 1977. Regulation of immunoglobulin expression in mouse myeloma cells. *Cold Spring Harbor Symp. Quant. Biol.* **41**:781.

Marshak-Rothstein, A., P. Fink, T. Gridley, D.H. Raulet, M.J. Bevan, and M.L. Gefter. 1979. Properties and applications of monoclonal antibodies directed against determinants of the Thy-1 locus. *J. Immunol.* **122**:2491.

Matus, A.I. and D.H. Taff-Jones. 1978. Morphology and molecular composition of isolated post-synaptic junctional structures. *Proc. R. Soc. London B* **203**:135.

Matus, A.I., B.B. Walters, and S. Mughal. 1975. Immunohistochemical demonstration of tubulin associated with microtubule and synaptic junctions in mammalian brain. *J. Neurocytol.* **4**:733.

Melchers, F., M. Potter, and N. Warner, eds. 1979. *Lymphocyte hybridomas.* Springer-Verlag, New York.

Milstein, C., K. Adetugbo, N.J. Cowan, G. Köhler, D.S. Secher, and C.D. Wilde. 1977. Somatic cell genetics of antibody-secreting cells: Studies of clonal diversification and analysis by cell fusion. *Cold Spring Harbor Symp. Quant. Biol.* **41:**793.

Mishell, B.B. and S.M. Shugi, eds. 1980. *Selected methods in cellular immunology.* Freeman, San Francisco.

Morita, K., R.A. North, and Y. Katayama. 1980. Evidence that substance P is a neurotransmitter in the myenteric plexus. *Nature* **287:**151.

Nabel, G., M. Fresno, A. Chessman, and H. Cantor. 1981. Use of cloned populations of mouse lymphocytes to analyze cellular differentiation. *Cell* **23:**19.

Nicoll, R.A., C. Schenker, and S.E. Leeman. 1980. Substance P as a transmitter candidate. *Annu. Rev. Biochem.* **3:**227.

Nishi, R. and D. Berg. 1979. Survival and development of ciliary ganglion neurones grown alone in tissue culture. *Nature* **277:**232.

Nossal, G. and J. Lederberg. 1958. Antibody production by single cells. *Nature* **181:**1419.

O'Sullivan, M.J., E. Gnemml, A.D. Simmonds, G. Chieregatti, E. Heyderman, J.W. Bridges, and V. Marks. 1979. A comparison of the ability of B-galactosidase and HRP enzyme-antibody conjugates to detect specific antibodies. *J. Immunol. Methods* **31:**247.

Parham, P. 1979. Purification of immunologically active HLA-A and -B antigens by a series of monoclonal antibody columns. *J. Biol. Chem.* **254:**8709.

Patterson, P.H. and L.L.Y. Chun. 1977. The induction of acetylcholine synthesis in primary cultures of dissociated rat sympathetic neurons. I. Effects of conditioned medium. *Dev. Biol.* **56:**263.

Potter, M. and F. Melchers, eds. 1978. *Curr. Top. Immunol. Microbiol.,* vol. 81.

Raff, M.C., K.L. Fields, S. Hakamori, R. Mirsky, R.M. Pruss, and J. Winter. 1979. Cell-type-specific markers for distinguishing and studying neurons and the major classes of glial cells in culture. *Brain Res.* **174:**283.

Richards, F.F., W.H. Konigsberg, R.W. Rosenstein, and J.M. Varga. 1975. On the specificity of antibodies. *Science* **187:**130.

Sanes, J.R. and Z.W. Hall. 1979. Antibodies that bind specifically to synaptic sites on muscle fiber basal lamina. *J. Cell Biol.* **83:**357.

Sanes, J.R., L.M. Marshall, and U.J. McMahan. 1978. Reinnervation of muscle fiber basal lamina after removal of myofibers. Differentiation of regenerating axons at original synaptic sites. *J. Cell Biol.* **78:**176.

Seidman, J., A. Leder, M. Nau, B. Norman, and P. Leder. 1978. Antibody diversity. *Science* **202:**11.

Sigal, N.H. and N.R. Klinman. 1978. The B-cell clonotype repertoire. *Adv. Immunol.* **26:**255.

Snyder, S.H. and R.B. Innis. 1979. Peptide neurotransmitters. *Annu. Rev. Biochem.* **48:**755.

Springer, T.A. 1980. Characterization of "jumping" and "lineage" antigens using xenogeneic rat monoclonal antibodies. In *Monoclonal Antibodies* (ed. R.H. Kennet, T.J. McKearn, and K.B. Bechtol), p. 185. Plenum Press, New York.

Stell, W., D. Marshak, T. Yamada, N. Brecha, and H. Karten. 1980. Peptides are in the eye of the beholder. *Trends Neurosci.* **3**:292.

Tonegawa, S., H. Sakano, R. Maki, A. Traunecker, G. Heinrich, W. Roeder, and Y. Kurosawa. 1981. Somatic reorganization of immunoglobulin genes during lymphocyte differentiation. *Cold Spring Harbor Symp. Quant. Biol.* **45**:839.

Tsuchiya, S., S. Yokoyama, O. Yoshie, and Y. Ono. 1980. Production of diphtheria antitoxin antibody in Epstein-Barr virus–induced lymphoblastoid cell lines. *J. Immunol.* **124**:1970.

van Vunakis, H. and J.J. Langone, eds. 1980. Immunochemical techniques. *Methods Enzymol.*, vol. 70.

Wood, J.G., R.W. Wallace, J.N. Whittaker, and W.Y. Cheung. 1980. Immunocytochemical localization of calmodulin and a heat-labile calmodulin binding protein (CaM-BP$_{80}$) in basal ganglia of mouse brain. *J. Cell Biol.* **84**:66.

Zurawski, V.R., Jr., E. Haber, and P.H. Black. 1978. Production of antibody to tetanus toxoid by continuous human lymphoblastoid cell lines. *Science* **199**:1439.

Monoclonal Antibodies Recognizing Subpopulations of Glial Cells in Mouse Cerebellum

MELITTA SCHACHNER, ILSE SOMMER, CAROL LAGENAUR, and JUTTA SCHNITZER

Department of Neurobiology
University of Heidelberg
Heidelberg, Federal Republic of Germany D-6900

• Our aim is to investigate cell-cell interactions in the developing cerebellum of normal mice and developmentally abnormal mutants. It seems important, therefore, to isolate individual cell populations at different developmental stages by immunoselective measures via antibodies to cell-surface components and to find and characterize markers to subsets of neural cell types to identify cell-lineage relationships and, hopefully, thereby reveal functional properties as well.

OLIGODENDROCYTE CELL-SURFACE MARKERS

• Four antibodies were raised against antigens, designated 01, 02, 03, and 04, that are expressed on the surfaces of oligodendrocytes (Schachner 1981; Sommer and Schachner 1981). They were produced by immunizing BALB/c mice with homogenized white matter from bovine corpus callosum and fusing their spleen cells with the myeloma NS1 (Galfre et al. 1977; Fazekas de St. Groth and Scheidegger 1980). The resultant hybridoma supernatants were screened by indirect immunofluorescence on both fresh-frozen tissue sections and cultured cells to enable detection of minor cell populations.

All antigens (01, 02, 03, and 04) were expressed on rat, mouse, chick, and human nervous systems. All four antibodies were IgM and were cytotoxic with complement. At limiting antibody dilutions, the processes of oligodendrocytes could be lysed and the cell bodies spared. In primary cultures of neonatal mouse nervous system (cerebellum, cerebrum, spinal cord, and optic nerve), all four antibodies stained the surfaces of cells that were positive for galactocerebroside (GC) and were negative for tetanus toxin, fibronectin, and glial fibrillary acidic protein (GFAP). In addition, 03 and 04 were expressed on the surfaces of cells that were negative for GC as well as for tetanus toxin, fibronectin, and GFAP. These cells had a very similar morphology to oligodendrocytes in electron micrographs of immunoperoxidase-stained cultured cells (G. Berg and M. Schachner, in prep.).

In fresh-frozen sections of adult mouse cerebellum, all the 0 antigens were detectable in white-matter tracts and in the granular layer. However, 02 and 03 were seen in GFAP-positive radial fibers in the molecular layer. 01, 02, and 03 seemed to be expressed in a fibrillar, GFAP-like pattern in fixed, cultured astrocytes from the cerebellum. 04 was also expressed on dorsal root ganglion neurons, especially after long periods in culture.

When neonatal cerebellum was dissociated with trypsin and stained in suspension for the presence of the four antigens, only the 03 and 04 antigens could be detected, whereas by postnatal day 7, antigens 01, 02, 03, and 04 were all expressed (Table 1).

Moreover, in primary cultures of fetal pons and cerebellum, expression of 03 and 04 antigens preceded that of 01 and 02. If such cultures were prepared from 7-day-old mice, the percentage of 03- and 04-antigen-positive but GC-negative cells was higher after 2 days in vitro than after 7, when nearly all of the 03- and 04-positive cells

Table 1

Properties of Oligodendrocyte-associated Antigens in the Cerebellum

	Antigens			
	01	02	03	04
Development				
Neonate (day 0)	−	−	+	+
Neonate (day 7)	+	+	+	+
Adult	+	+	+	+
Cell types with antigen in culture				
Galactocerebroside +/− oligodendrocyte	+	+	+	+
Galactocerebroside +/− oligodendrocytelike cell	−	−	+	+
Astrocyte	+	+	+	−
Sensory neuron	−	−	−	+
Adult cerebellum				
White matter	+	+	+	+
Bergmann glia	(0)	+	+	−

were also positive for GC, 01, and 02. These cells had, in general, many fine cellular processes.

To determine whether or not the 03- and 04-positive cells were precursors of 01-, 02-, 03-, 04-, and GC-positive oligodendrocytes, freshly isolated cell suspensions from 7-day-old mouse cerebellum were selectively depleted of 01-positive cells either by complement-dependent cytotoxicity or by coating polyacrylamide iron-cored beads with monoclonal anti-01 antibody; these beads were mixed with the cell suspensions, and then beads plus specific cells were removed with a magnet (D. Meier and M. Schachner, unpubl.). The remaining 01- and 02-negative cells were then cultured and stained for the presence of 03 and 04 antigens by reacting with 04 antibody directly coupled to rhodamine. One or two days later, the cells were stained with anti-01 antibody conjugated to fluorescein. 01-Antigen-positive cells that had internalized rhodamine could be seen, suggesting that they were originally stained with 04 antibodies. These observations indicate that 04-positive cells are precursors to 01- and GC-positive cells.

ASTROCYTE CYTOPLASMIC MARKERS

• Two monoclonal antibodies were raised that recognized astrocytes C1 and M1.

C1

Monoclonal anti-C1 antibody (I. Sommer et al., in prep.) was produced by immunizing mice with bovine corpus callosum white matter and fusing their spleen cells with the myeloma NS1. It reacts with an intracellular antigen present in mouse but no other species. Indirect immunofluorescence on fixed cells showed that C1 was expressed in cultured astrocytes and fibroblasts. In fresh-frozen sections from 11-day mouse embryos, the antigen was seen in radially orientated processes in the telencephalon, pons, and pituitary and retinal anlage. In neonatal cerebellum, Bergmann glia and astrocytes of prospective white matter stain with anti-C1. In the adult cerebellum and retina, C1 antigen was restricted to Bergmann glia and Müller cells and was absent from GFAP-positive astrocytes in other parts of the brain. Ependymal cells and cells of large blood vessels were also positive for C1. C1 antigen was not detectable in radial glia or other cerebellar astrocytes in the neurologically mutant mice staggerer (sg), reeler (rl), or weaver (wv) but was present in the ependyma and large blood vessels of these mice (Tables 2 and 3).

M1

Monoclonal anti-M1 antibody was produced from a fusion of NS1 myeloma cells with spleen cells from rats that had been immunized with crude membranes from early postnatal mouse cerebella (Lagenaur et al. 1980). In cerebellar cultures it recognized an intracellular antigen expressed in a proportion of GFAP-positive astrocytes.

In sections from 7-day-old mouse cerebellum, M1 antigen was present in astrocytes of prospective white matter and internal granular layer, and at day 10 it was also seen in Bergmann glia. In adult brain, M1 was only detected in white-matter astrocytes but could no longer be detected in Bergmann glia or granular-layer astrocytes. However, in mutant mice (st, rl, and wv) M1 persisted in Bergmann glia in adult brain (Tables 2 and 3).

M1 and C1 antigens therefore seem specific for different subpopulations of astrocytes and may be useful markers for studying astrocyte maturation and differentiation.

Table 2

Localization of Antigens in Neural Cell Types of Mouse

Antigen	Embryonic CNS	Early postnatal cerebellum	Adult CNS	Mutants (≥17 days old) (sg, rl, wv)
C1	radial fibers	Bergmann glia; astrocytes in prospective white matter	Bergmann glia; retinal Müller cells; ependyma	Bergmann glia negative[1]; ependyma[2]
M1	negative	Bergmann glia; astrocytes in prospective white matter	astrocytes in cerebellar white matter and retinal ganglion cell layer	Bergmann glia[1]; astrocytes in granular layer[1] and white matter[2]
Vimentin	radial fibers; ventricular cells	Bergmann glia; astrocytes in prospective white matter; ependyma	all astrocytes; ependyma	all astrocytes[2]; ependyma[2]
GFAP	negative	more mature astrocytes	all astrocytes	all astrocytes[2]

[1]Abnormal.
[2]Normal.

Table 3

Astrocyte-associated Antigen Appearance in Cerebellums of Normal and Mutant Mice

	C1	M1
Embryo		
Radial fibers	+	−
Early postnatal		
Bergmann glia	+	+
Astrocytes in white matter	+	+
Normal adult		
Bergmann glia	+	−
Astrocytes in granular layer	−	−
Astrocytes in white matter	−	+
Ependyma	+	−
Mutant mice (sg, rl, wv)		
Bergmann glia	−	+
Astrocytes in granular layer	−	+
Astrocytes in white matter	−	+
Ependyma	+	−

REFERENCES

Berg, G. and M. Schachner. 1981. Immunoelectron microscopic identification of 0-antigen bearing oligodendroglial cells in vitro. *Cell Tissue Res.* (in press).

Fazekas de St. Groth, S. and D. Scheidegger. 1980. Production of monoclonal antibodies: Strategy and tactics. *J. Immunol. Methods* **35**:1.

Galfre, G., S.C. Howe, C. Milstein, G.W. Butcher, and J.C. Howard. 1977. Antibodies to major histocompatibility antigens produced by hybrid cell lines. *Nature* **266**:550.

Lagenaur, C., I. Sommer, and M. Schachner. 1980. Subclass of astroglia in mouse cerebellum recognized by monoclonal antibody. *Dev. Biol.* **79**:367.

Schachner, M., S.K. Kim, and R. Zehnle. 1981. Developmental expression in central and peripheral nervous system of oligodendrocyte cell surface antigens (0 antigens) recognized by monoclonal antibodies. *Dev. Biol.* **83**:328.

Sommer, I. and M. Schachner. 1981. Monoclonal antibodies (01 to 04) to oligodendrocyte cell surfaces: An immunocytological study in the central nervous system. *Dev. Biol.* **83**:311.

Conventional Antibodies to Intermediate Filament Subunit Proteins Show the Cell-type Specificity of 10-nm Filaments

KAY L. FIELDS and SHU-HUI YEN

Departments of Neurology and Pathology
Albert Einstein College of Medicine
Bronx, New York 10461

• Ten-nm filaments, intermediate in size between microtubules (25 nm) and actin filaments (6 nm), are present in large amounts in the nervous system but are in other tissues as well. So far, five different types of intermediate filaments (IF) have been described, as summarized in Table 1.

One or more of these classes of IFs exists in most cell types. Neurofilaments, tonofilaments, and glial filaments are specific to neurons, epithelial cells, and astrocytes, respectively, whereas vimentin has been demonstrated to be present in a wide variety of cell types in addition to fibroblasts, especially in embryonic and cultured tissue. Desmin has been found in fibroblasts as well as muscle.

Table 1
Five Types of Intermediate Filaments

	Vimentin	Desmin	Tono-filaments	Glial filaments	Neuro-filaments
Defined in	fibroblasts	muscle	epithelia	fibrous astrocytes	axons
No. of different polypeptide subunits	1	1	4−9	1	3
m.w. ($\times 10^{-3}$)	55−58	55−53	40−70	49−51	~ 210, 160, 68

Although work with a monoclonal antibody suggests that all IFs have a common antigenic part as well as distinctive parts (see Pruss et al., this volume), with conventional rabbit antisera the differences between various IFs have been immunodominant. We have used antisera to vimentin (Hynes and Destree 1978), to the 49-kilodalton (49K) glial filament subunit polypeptide and to the largest (210K) neurofilament polypeptide in order to establish the cell-type specificity of each serum, using cells in tissue culture and tissue sections of the central and peripheral nervous systems (CNS and PNS) (Yen and Fields 1981). For the first time, we have shown that Schwann cells and astrocytes have vimentin filaments and that the neurofilament antiserum stains cultured neurons specifically. In addition, we find some astrocyte-filament-like antigen far out in sciatic nerve.

ANTISERA

• IFs were purified from white matter of human autopsy brains, and samples were run on preparative (SDS-polyacrylamide gel electrophoresis) gels. The 210K neurofilament band and the 49K band were cut out of the gel, emulsified with Freund's complete adjuvant, and injected into different rabbits. After boosting, the antisera were tested using a rocket immunoelectrophoresis method with detergents (Mahadik et al. 1980) to establish specificity, i.e., with which cytoskeletal proteins (separated on SDS gels) did they react.

The anti-49K serum gives a precipitation line with the 49K band from SDS gels but not with 210K, 160K, or 68K proteins. Anti-210K does not react with the 49K protein but precipitates 210K, 160K, and 68K proteins by reacting with common, but neurofilament-specific, determinants.

The other antiserum used in this study was an anti-vimentin serum of Hynes and Destree (1978) that was raised against the 58K polypeptide from the cytoskeleton preparation of NIL-8 hamster fibroblasts.

RESULTS

Anti-210K and Neurofilaments

• Fresh-frozen cryostat sections of adult rat cerebellum and sciatic nerve were examined for staining with anti-210K. Staining was seen in sciatic nerve in the axoplasm of the large, myelinated axons (Fig. 1a). The myelin sheath, Schwann cells, and connective tissue were all negative. In cerebellum, fiber tracts stained strongly and positive processes were seen in the granular layer. Bergmann glia, other glial cells, blood vessels, and pia were all negative.

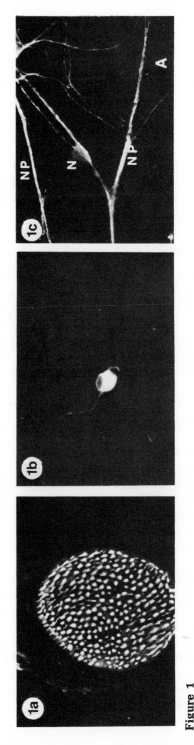

Figure 1

Anti-210K serum stains axons in sciatic nerve and the cytoplasm of cultured neurons. (*a*) Cryostat section of rat sciatic nerve incubated with anti-210K serum (1:50) and goat anti-rabbit-immunoglobulin–fluorescein (1:60). The fluorescence is confined to axons. Magnification, 141×. (*b*) A dissociated neuron from rat dorsal root ganglion binds anti-210K serum (1:300), detected with a rhodamine-labeled goat anti–rabbit IgG (1:150). In this field there are four Schwann cells that do not stain with this serum and are invisible. Magnification, 326×. (*c*) Neuronal processes (NP) of cerebellar cells in culture bind anti-210K serum (1:100), whereas small granule cell neurons (N) or the background astrocytes (A; invisible) fail to stain. Cells in culture for 8 days (with added FUdR), fixed and stained as in *b*. Magnification, 534×. (Reprinted, with permission, from Yen and Fields 1981.)

In primary cultures of dorsal root ganglia, about 80% of the neurons stained with anti-210K in the cell soma and processes. Schwann cells and fibroblasts were negative (Fig. 1b). In cerebellar cultures, some of the neuronal cells stained, but astrocytes, fibroblasts, oligodendroglia, and most granule cell neurons did not (Fig. 1c).

Electron microscopy

At the ultrastructural level, the anti-210K serum could be seen to bind to filaments inside neurons, but not astrocytes, by immunoperoxidase staining of rat cortex. Neuronal plasma membranes and outer mitochondrial membranes adjacent to the filaments also showed some staining, but the significance of this is unclear.

Anti-49K and Glial Filaments

In cryostat sections and cultures of the CNS, astrocytes stained with anti-49K. However, staining was also seen in rat sciatic nerve cryostat sections (Fig. 2a), an observation that is in apparent conflict with previous reports. In longitudinal sections of sciatic nerve, the staining was seen as single fibers or processes or as groups of long, thin elements parallel to the myelinated axons. This staining could be adsorbed out with cytoskeletal preparations from astrocytes but not from fibroblasts. Thus, peripheral nerve contains an antigen that cross-reacts with glial IFs. Whether or not a 49K protein in sciatic nerve preparations accounts for this staining is not yet known, but all anti-GFAP (anti−glial fibrillary acidic protein) sera tested detected the same elements. They occur in rat, mouse, and cat sciatic nerve.

To decide what cell type was staining, the sciatic nerves of adult rats were transected and the distal portion examined 1 week to 8 weeks later. Staining with anti-49K was seen to increase dramatically in the cut nerves and persist long after neurofilament antigen and degenerating myelin had disappeared. The 49K-like antigen may well be in Schwann cells, which are known to proliferate in response to injury.

If tissue sections of sciatic nerves from rats younger than 11 days were tested, no anti-49K or anti-GFAP staining was seen, in agreement with previous results with cultured cells from neonatal animals. However, R. Mirsky (pers. comm.) has tested cultures of 11- or 12-day-old rat sciatic nerve and found that a few cells did stain for GFAP and the Schwann cell surface marker Ran-1. Jessen and Mirsky (1980) also found GFAP-positive cells in the enteric plexus of the gut, both in frozen sections and in cultures. We favor the hypothesis that the antigen in gut and sciatic nerve comes from similar or closely related cells (Fields 1980).

Anti-58K and Vimentin Filaments

Fibroblasts and Schwann cells both stained with anti-58K sera in
sciatic nerve cryostat sections (Fig. 2b) and in cultures of sciatic
nerve or peripheral ganglia (Fig. 3a). Filaments inside Schwann cells
had been seen by electron microscopy, but positive staining with
vimentin antisera has not been shown before.

In cryostat sections of the adult rat cerebellum, Bergmann glial
fibers and fibrous astrocytes in white matter stained, whereas GFAP-
positive astrocytes in the granular layer failed to stain with anti-
vimentin. In culture, most, if not all, GFAP-positive astrocytes were
vimentin-positive. With further development in vivo, some astrocytes
may stop making vimentin.

The intermediate filaments of cultured astrocytes were characterized biochemically (Chiu et al. 1980). When cytoskeletal preparations
were run on SDS gels, the major bands were at 58K, 50K, and 42K
plus histone proteins. Fibroblasts had a similar profile, except they
were missing the 50K band. Peptide mapping showed that the 42K
band in both preparations was closely related to muscle actin. The
58K protein of rat astrocytes or fibroblasts gave indistinguishable
maps from the 58K vimentin band of control NIL-8 cells. The 58K,
50K, and 42K maps are easily distinguished from each other.

Both vimentin- and astrocyte-filament staining were shown to
form coils around the nucleus in response to colchicine treatment of
cultured cells (Fig. 3b). It is not known whether astrocytes have two

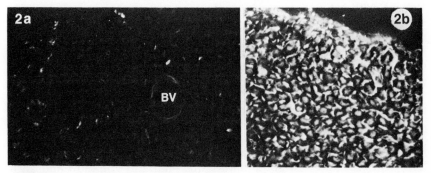

Figure 2
The patterns of staining of sciatic nerve by anti-49K and anti-58K sera are
different. Cross sections of nerve stained with (a) anti-49K serum (1:50) show
a few elements outside the myelinated axons, whereas (b) anti-58K serum
(1:75) detects elements around the periphery of each myelin sheath. Magnification, 324×. This anti-58K serum (Hynes and Destree 1978) shows natural
antibodies (present in the preimmunization bleeding) that bind to the axons;
other anti-58K rabbit sera did not have these. (Reprinted, with permission,
from Yen and Fields 1981.)

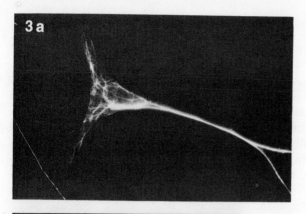

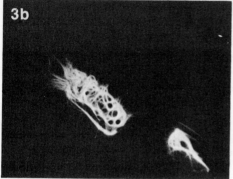

Figure 3
(a) Schwann cells in culture have filamentous
staining with anti-58K serum (1:75) (but not with
anti−210K, anti−49K, or anti−keratin filament
sera). Magnification, 620×. (b) Astrocytes stain
with anti-49K and anti-58K sera, and both antigens
coil in response to colchicine treatment (18 hr);
shown here are two astrocytes stained with anti-
49K (1:50). Magnification, 407×. (Reprinted, with
permission, from Yen and Fields 1981.)

filament systems, or whether individual filaments in astrocytes contain both 58K and 50K subunits. Monoclonal anti-vimentin and anti-
GFAP may be necessary to resolve this question.

Conventional rabbit antisera have been very useful in distinguishing the different classes of IFs. Luckily, the insoluble and nearly
inseparable subunit proteins were good immunogens after separation
on SDS gels. These antisera have shown that neurofilaments are
confined to neurons; glial filaments are in astrocytes and some peripheral nerve cells; and vimentin is found in fibroblasts, Schwann
cells, and astrocytes. Hopefully, a set of monoclonal antibodies to the

filament subunits will confirm these conclusions as well as provide information about the separate neurofilament proteins and the relationships of the subunits to one another.

REFERENCES

Chiu, F.-C., W.T. Norton, and K.L. Fields. 1981. The cytoskeleton of primary astrocytes in culture contains actin, glial fibrillary acidic protein, and the fibroblast-type filament protein, vimentin. *J. Neurochem.* (in press).

Fields, K.L. 1980. The study of Schwann cells using antigenic markers. *Trends Neurosci.* **3:**236.

Hynes, R.O. and A.T. Destree. 1978. 10 nm filaments in normal and transformed cells. *Cell* **13:**151.

Jessen, K.R. and R. Mirsky. 1980. Glial cells in the enteric nervous system contain glial fibrillary acidic protein. *Nature* **286:**286.

Mahadik, S.P., A. Korenovsky, Y. Huang, L. Gray, and M.M. Rapport. 1980. Synaptic membrane antigen, detection and characterization. *J. Neurosci. Methods* **2:**169.

Yen, S.-H. and K.L. Fields. 1981. Antibodies to neurofilament, glial filament and fibroblast intermediate filament proteins bind to different cell types of the nervous system. *J. Cell Biol.* **88:**115.

Surface-membrane Markers as Probes for Neuronal Development

YOHEVED BERWALD-NETTER and ANNETTE KOULAKOFF

Biochimie Cellulaire, Collège de France
Paris, France 75231

FRANCOIS COURAUD

INSERM U-172, Faculté de Médecine Nord
Marseille, France 13326

• A necessary prerequisite for the study of neuronal ontogeny is the availability of markers that can distinguish neurons from other cells at early developmental stages. We have used three surface markers, which in vitro interact selectively with fetal neurons, in order to determine the schedule of appearance and accumulation of presumptive neuroblasts and neurons in the mouse nervous system developing in vivo. The markers are:

1. Tetanus toxin (TT): It binds to long-chain gangliosides of the G1b series (van Heyningen 1963), which are present in brain of various vertebrates; their proportion in the central nervous system (CNS) of mice and rats increases considerably between 15 and 20 days of gestation (Irwin et al. 1980). The neuronal association of TT-binding sites was indicated by a high toxin-fixing capacity to synaptic membranes and to tissue cultures of fetal mouse brain and spinal cord. Subsequently, it was shown that TT can be used in vitro as a neuronal marker, by selective surface-labeling of neurons in cultures of peripheral and central nervous tissue (Dimpfel et al. 1977; Mirsky et al. 1978). The schedule of appearance in vivo of TT-binding cells has not been determined.

2. Rabbit anti-neuroblastoma (anti-NB) antisera, raised against the differentiated C1300 cell line N-18 or T-28: These sera label the same cells that bind TT in indirect in vitro immunofluorescence assays (Fig. 1). Quantitative adsorptions indicated the presence of the corresponding antigens in early fetal brain and, in a much higher amount, in the adult (Berwald-

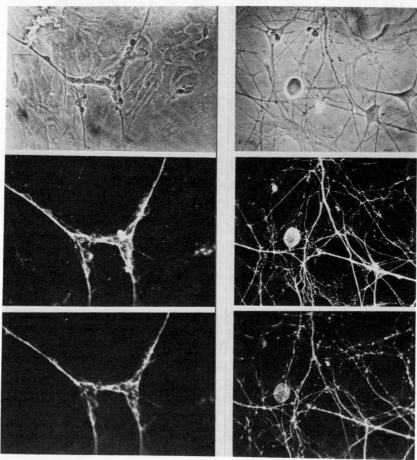

Figure 1
Double immunofluorescence labeling of mouse brain cells in culture (*left*) and of cultured mouse DRG (*right*) with anti-NB antibodies and TT. (*Top*) Phase contrast; (*middle*) anti-NB labeling (revealed by goat anti–rabbit Ig/ tetramethyl rhodmine isothiocyanate [TRITC]); (*bottom*) TT labeling (revealed by horse anti–tetanus IgG/fluorescein isothiocyanate [FITC]). The cultures were labeled unfixed at room temperature, with 3 rinses following each reagent. They were scanned for fluorescence after brief drying and alcohol fixation. Note overlap of labeling, by both reagents, of cells with neuronal morphology and the lack of labeling of astrocytes and Schwann cells.

      Netter and Koulakoff 1979). Neither the nature nor the function of the antigen(s) recognized is known.
3. Scorpion toxin (ScT), purified from the venom of the African scorpion *Androctonus a. Hector*: It binds to receptors on voltage-dependent Na^+ channels of excitable cells (reviewed by Rochat et al. 1979; Catterall 1980).

The toxin binds with high affinity (K_d = 0.1–1.0 nM) to brain synaptosomal preparations and to cultured C1300 neuroblastoma cells. Since the binding is voltage-dependent, depolarized or damaged cells bind very little toxin specifically. Moreover, the toxin can be ^{125}I-labeled to a high specific activity (700–1000 Ci/mmole) without a change in its binding properties. In earlier studies in vitro, we have shown (Berwald-Netter et al. 1980) that at ^{125}I-labeled ScT concentrations of 0.05–20 nM, a high binding is seen in cultures enriched for neurons, whereas in cultures of CNS glia with no visible neurons, the binding is close to background values. ScT can thus be a useful tool for studying excitable cells at early developmental stages when electrophysiology is difficult due to the small size and fragility of the cells and when cell identification based on morphology is deceptive. Furthermore, the function of the molecule to which ScT binds is known.

RESULTS

• To examine the development of cells that get labeled by anti-NB serum and by TT (Berwald-Netter et al. 1980), cells were mechanically dissociated from whole brain of mice of various ages and double-stained with the two reagents. In preparations from 10-day embryos, close to 3% of cells stained with both TT and anti-NB, increasing to about 60% in fetuses of 18 or 19 days (Fig. 2). At all ages, nearly all cells that were labeled with TT were also labeled with anti-NB, and about 10% of the total number of cells were NB-positive and TT-negative. These cells are thought to be neuronal precursors destined to become TT-positive. To verify this hypothesis, sorting out of the cells is currently being attempted.

The timing of the appearance and the pattern of accumulation of TT-binding cells (TTBC) in different parts of the nervous system (Fig. 3) differs from that seen in whole brain (Fig. 4). In cerebellum and spinal cord, the percentage of TTBC falls and then rises again. The fall is probably due to a developmental asynchrony in the accumulation of TTBC and of precursor cells lacking TT receptors, as well as to a "morphogenetic death" (Prestige 1970) of cell subpopulations. This phenomenon, particularly well documented for the ventral horns of spinal cord (Harris Flanagan 1968; Hamburger 1975), is a common feature of many embryonic tissues. Glia are thought to represent only a small proportion of total cells at this stage, since most glial cells develop postnatally. Labeling of dorsal root ganglion (DRG) cells follows a sigmoid curve similar to that seen in whole brain, except that the slope of the curve is somewhat steeper and the maximal TTBC ratio attained (day-18 fetuses) is higher (~ 80% in DRG com-

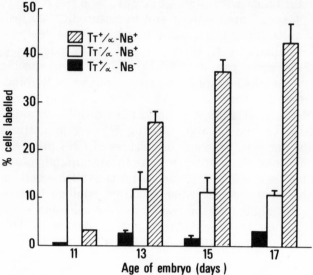

Figure 2
The proportion of mouse brain cells binding anti-NB, or
TT, or both in doubly labeled cell suspensions at different fetal ages. Cells were dissociated mechanically in
$Ca^{++}Mg^{++}$-free PBS. They were treated sequentially at 4°C
with TT, antitoxin–horse IgG/FITC, rabbit anti-NB, and
goat anti–rabbit Ig/TRITC. Three washes followed each
treatment. All antibodies were preadsorbed with mouse
fetal brain cells. Controls consisted of cells treated with
the labeled antibodies only. (TT) Tetanus toxin; (α-NB)
anti-NB.

pared with 57 ± 5% in whole brain). The time of emergence and the
profiles of accumulation of TTBC in the various parts of mouse
nervous system studied (Koulakoff et al., in prep.) are temporally
consistent with neuronal birthday data and accumulation rhythm of
postmitotic neurons determined by tritiated thymidine incorporation
(Angevine 1970; Sidman 1970 and references therein).

For ScT binding, a different assay system was used (Berwald-
Netter et al. 1981). Cell suspensions derived from mouse brains at
different stages of prenatal development were examined by radioassay for the presence of toxin receptors (Fig. 4). The onset of detectable
^{125}I-labeled ScT binding lags behind the appearance of anti-NB- and
TT-binding cells by 2 days and was first demonstrated on 12-day
embryos. Binding increases slowly until embryonic day 15 and then

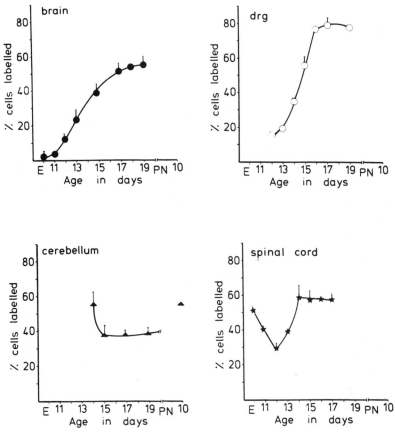

Figure 3
Evolution of TT-binding cells in different regions of mouse nervous system. Cell preparation and labeling were as described in the legend to Fig. 2. (E) Embryo days; (PN) postnatal days.

increases rapidly (Fig. 5). At all stages, the ScT binds with high affinity (K_d = 0.1–0.5 nM) to a single class of noninteracting sites (shown by linear Scatchard plots). The binding is voltage-dependent.

It is not known from these binding assays whether the toxin binds to all cells or to a subpopulation. However, as mentioned above, ScT-binding assays done on cultured fetal mouse brain cells showed that only cultures of neurons that also bind TT express high-affinity binding sites for ScT. Therefore, the mean number and density of sites, determined initially per cell, was recalculated per TT-binding cell, the proportion of which was established in parallel for each binding assay done. The mean number of ScT-binding sites per

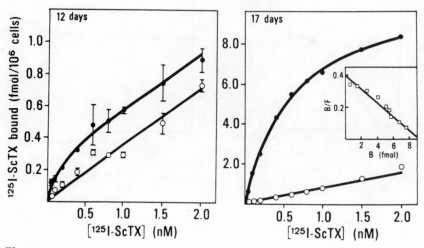

Figure 4
Binding of ^{125}I-labeled ScT to dissociated fetal mouse brain cells. (•) Total
binding; (o) nonspecific binding (in presence of excess of native toxin); (□)
Scatchard plot of specific binding. Binding was done at 37°C for 30 min. The
cells (dissociated as for Fig. 2) were suspended in Na$^+$-free incubation buffer
containing 140 mM choline chloride to ensure isotonicity without depolarization. Unbound toxin was removed by three cold washes, and toxin bound to
cell pellets was counted in a γ-scintillation counter.

TT-positive cell is 1040 (or 4.2/μm^2) at 12 embryonic days and increases to 33,900 (or 136/μm^2) by fetal day 19. Since there is practical-
ly no difference in the mean cell diameters at the earliest and latest
times examined and since there is only a twofold difference between
the smallest and the biggest cell diameters, it follows that the high
density of binding sites noted at later stages involves a high proportion of cells with high receptor density. It may thus be an indication
of a qualitative change in the functioning of neurons and correspond
to a phase when many start emitting action potentials. Indeed, the
ScT density we determined on brain cells at 16 fetal days or later is
very close to, or higher than, the estimated density of Na$^+$ channels
on excitable, nonmyelinated nerves (Ritchie and Rogart 1977).

    Part of this time-course study was repeated in vitro on cells
derived from 15-day fetal brains and examined with time in culture.
Again, the number of ScT-binding sites per cell increases with time;
there was no change in the binding affinity, and the binding was

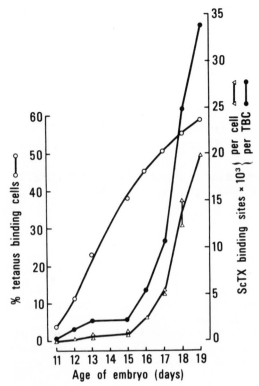

Figure 5
Quantitative evolution of ScT-binding sites
on fetal mouse brain cells developing in vivo.
The number of toxin-binding sites was derived from saturable binding curves as in Fig.
4. The data were calculated either per cell (Δ)
or per TT-binding cell (TBC) (●). The proportion of TBC at each age is shown (o).

voltage-dependent. Neurite elaboration preceded the steep increase in
toxin binding by about 48 hours. Therefore, the higher number of
binding sites per cell could not be accounted for by an increase in
surface area due to neurite extension and must have resulted from an
actual increase in binding sites per μm^2.

In conclusion, we have shown that ligands are available that
allow a direct identification of viable neuroblasts and/or neurons at
very early stages of mammalian CNS organogenesis. The visible abundance of surface components binding TT or neuron-specific antibodies can be exploited for selective cell sorting. ScT high-affinity
binding to the Na^+-channel-associated receptors can be used as a

quantitative index of neuronal differentiation and maturation. Together with other markers described in this volume, these ligands provide valuable tools in the study of nervous system development.

ACKNOWLEDGMENTS

• The authors acknowledge the generous gifts of TT and TT antibodies from Dr. B. Bizzini, as well as of purified ScT from Dr. H. Rochat.

We also acknowledge the financial support by DGRST, INSERM (ATP 81.79.113), CNRS (ATP 09-4-192), and Ligue Nationale Française contre le Cancer.

REFERENCES

Angevine, J.B. 1970. Critical cellular events in the shaping of neural centers. In The neurosciences second study program (ed. F.O. Schmitt and T. Melnechuk), p. 62. Rockefeller University Press, New York.

Berwald-Netter, Y. and A. Koulakoff. 1979. Neuronal surface antigenic markers revealed by rabbit anti-mouse C1300 neuroblastoma sera. In Seventh Meeting of the International Society for Neurochemistry, Jerusalem, p. 232. (Abstr.)

Berwald-Netter, Y., N. Martin-Moutot, A. Koulakoff, and F. Couraud. 1981. Na+-channel associated scorpion toxin receptor sites as probes for neuronal evolution in vivo and in vitro. Proc. Natl. Acad: Sci. 78:1245.

Berwald-Netter, Y., B. Bizzini, F. Couraud, A. Koulakoff, and N. Martin-Moutot. 1980. Three neurone-specific surface markers as probes for neuronal evolution in vivo and in vitro. Neurosci. Lett. (Suppl.) 5:311.

Catterall, W.A. 1980. Neurotoxins that act on voltage-sensitive sodium channels in excitable membranes. Annu. Rev. Pharmacol. Toxicol. 20:15.

Dimpfel, W., R.T.C. Huang, and E. Haberman. 1977. Gangliosides in nervous tissue cultures and binding of 125I-labelled tetanus toxin—A neuronal marker. J. Neurochem. 29:329.

Hamburger, V. 1975. Cell death in the development of the lateral column of the chick embryo. J. Comp. Neurol. 160:535.

Harris Flanagan, E. 1968. Differentiation and degeneration in the motor horn of the foetal mouse. J. Morphol. 129:281.

Irwin, L.N., D.B. Michael, and C.C. Irwin. 1980. Ganglioside patterns of fetal rat and mouse brain. J. Neurochem. 34:1527.

Mirsky, R., L.M.B. Wendon, P. Black, C. Stolkin, and D. Bray. 1978. Tetanus toxin: A cell surface marker for neurons in culture. Brain Res. 148:251.

Prestige, M.C. 1970. Differentiation, degeneration and the role of the periphery: Quantitative considerations. In The neurosciences second study program (ed. F.O. Schmitt and T. Melnechuk), p. 73. Rockefeller University Press, New York.

Ritchie, J.M. and R.B. Rogart. 1977. Density of sodium channels in mammalian myelinated nerve fibers and the nature of the axonal membrane under the myelin sheath. *Proc. Natl. Acad. Sci.* **74:**211.

Rochat, H., P. Bernard, and F. Couraud. 1979. Scorpion toxins: Chemistry and mode of action. *Adv. Cytopharmacol.* **3:**325.

Sidman, R.L. 1970. Cell proliferation, migration, and interaction in the developing mammalian central nervous system. In *The neurosciences second study program* (ed. F.O. Schmitt and T. Melnechuk), p. 100. Rockefeller University Press, New York.

van Heyningen, W.E. 1963. The fixation of tetanus toxin, strychnine, serotonin and other substances by ganglioside. *J. Gen. Microbiol.* **31:**375.

Monoclonal Antibody to the NG2 Marker

WILLIAM STALLCUP, JOEL LEVINE, and WILLIAM RASCHKE

The Salk Institute
San Diego, California 92138

• Of the wide range of stable cell lines derived from the rat central nervous system (CNS), some have neuronal properties, some have glial properties, and others have properties of both neurons and glia. Those classified as neuronal have three or four of the following characteristics:

1. They exhibit regenerative action potentials.
2. They express the neuron-specific antigens N1, N2, and N3, which were originally defined by antisera to two cell lines, B35 and B103, which had been classified as neuronal (Stallcup and Cohn 1976).
3. They have voltage-sensitive sodium channels, demonstrable by veratridine treatment (veratridine, which is known to open voltage-sensitive sodium channels, increases sodium uptake into excitable cells).
4. They have voltage-dependent potassium channels, which can be demonstrated by rubidium efflux studies (Arner and Stallcup 1981).
5. They do not express the glia-specific antigens G1 and G2, which were originally defined by rabbit antisera to cell lines C6B and B9, which were thought to be of glial origin.

Other cell lines can be classified as glial since they express the glial markers G1 and/or G2 on their surfaces and show none of the neuronal characteristics.

There is a third major group of cell lines that cannot be classified unambiguously as either neuronal or glial since they have properties of both cell types (see Table 1):

Table 1
Summary of Neuronal and Glial Properties

| Cell lines | Electrical properties | | | Antigens | | | | | |
	action potential[1]	Na⁺ channel[2]	K⁺ channel[3]	N1, N2, N3[2]	G1, G2[2]	N4	N5	NG1	NG2
Group 1 — neurons									
B11	+	+		+	−	+	−	−	−
B35	+	+	−	+	−	+	−	−	−
B50	+	+	+	+	−	−	−	−	−
B103	+	+	+	+	−	+	−	−	−
B104	+	+	−	+	−	+	−	−	−
XKM		+	−	+	−	+	−	−	−
XKC		+	+	+	−	+	−	−	−
ZKC		+	+	+	−	−	−	−	−
SW16		+	+	+	−	+	−	−	−
CK2D		+	+	+	−	+	−	−	−
Group 2 — pseudoneurons									
B19	−	+	+	−	+	+	+	−	+
B82	−	+	+	−	+	+	+	−	+
B108	−	+	+	−	+	+	+	+	+

Group 3 — pseudoglia									
(A) B49	−	−	+	−	+	−	−	−	+
B111	−	−	+	−	+	−	−	−	+
C6	−	−	+	−	+	−	−	−	+
βHC	−	−	+	−	+	−	−	−	+
(B) B9	−	−	+	−	+	−	−	+	−
BE11	−	−	+	−	+	−	−	+	−
B28	−	−	−	−	+	−	−	−	−
Group 4 — glia									
B15	−	−	−	−	+	−	−	−	−
B23	−	−	−	−	−	−	−	−	−
B27	−	−	−	−	+	−	−	−	−
B90	−	−	−	−	+	−	−	−	−
B92	−	−	−	−	+	−	−	−	−
βCFA	−	−	−	−	−	−	−	−	−
3T3	−	−	−	−	−	−	−	−	−

[1]Schubert et al. (1974).
[2]Stallcup and Cohn (1976); Bulloch et al. (1977).
[3]Arner and Stallcup (1980).

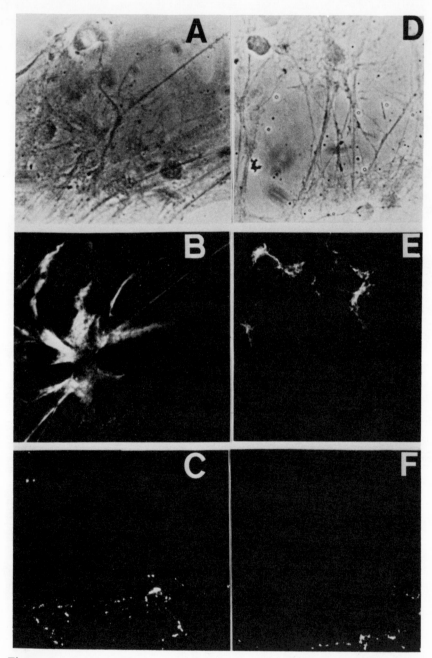

Figure 1

Doublelabeling in primary cultures of rat brain. Field 1: Three-week-old culture of 15-day embryonic rat brain; (A) phase; (B) anti-GFAP (fluorescein); (C) anti-NG2 (rhodamine). NG2⁺ cells were never costained with anti-GFAP. Field 2: Three-week-old culture of 15-day embryonic rat brain; (D) phase; (E) anti-GC (fluorescein); (F) anti-NG2 (rhodamine). NG2⁺ cells were never costained with anti-GC.

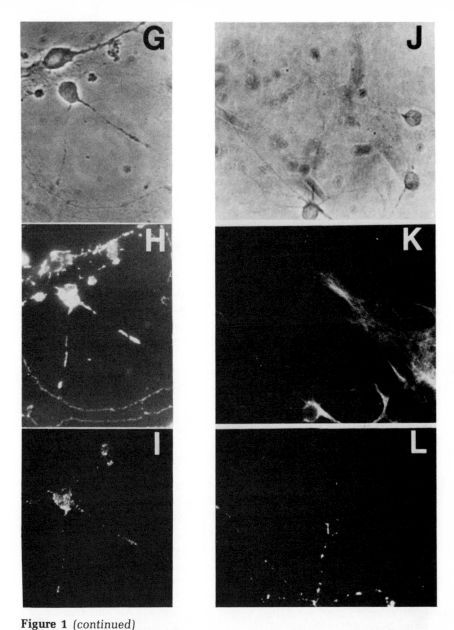

Figure 1 *(continued)*
Field 3: Three-week-old culture of 15-day embryonic rat brain; (G) phase; (H) tetanus toxin (TT) (fluorescein); (I) anti-NG2 (rhodamine). NG2$^+$ cells were often costained with TT. However, the majority of TT$^+$ cells (i.e., neurons) were not stained by anti-NG2. Field 4: Five-day-old culture of 4-day postnatal rat cerebellum; (J) phase; (K) anti-GFAP (fluorescein); (L) anti-NG2 (rhodamine). NG2$^+$ cells were often costained with anti-GFAP, in contrast to the results with 15-day embryonic brain. Anti-NG2 is not a general label for astrocytes, however; note the GFAP$^+$ cell in K that is not labeled by anti-NG2 in L.

1. They fail to exhibit regenerative action potentials.
2. They do not express N1, N2, or N3.
3. They express G1 and/or G2.
4. They have voltage-dependent potassium channels and some also have voltage-dependent sodium channels (Arner and Stallcup 1981).

One such cell line is B49, which has voltage-dependent potassium channels, typical of neurons, but which expresses G1 and G2 antigens, typical of glial cells. This cell line was used to immunize rabbits and mice to raise antisera that might detect antigens on a defined cell type in the nervous system. Whole B49 cells were injected intravenously into rabbits and mice, and the resultant antisera were adsorbed with two of the neuronal cell lines (Wilson et al. 1981).

Radioimmunoassay (RIA) showed that of 30 cell lines derived from rat and mouse CNS, only 7 reacted with the antisera (see Table 1). Interestingly, all of these cell lines were in the "ambiguous" category, having properties of both neurons and glia. Thus, the antiserum was named anti-NG2.

The next step was to find out whether these tumor-cell lines were expressing an inappropriate mixture of characteristics because they were neoplastic or whether there were cells in the normal nervous system with such mixed characteristics. By RIA, crude homogenates of rat brain were shown to express the NG2 antigen. Primary cultures of fetal and neonatal brain were examined for expression of NG2, galactocerebroside (GC) (Raff et al. 1978), glial fibrillary acidic protein (GFAP) (Bignami et al. 1972), and tetanus-toxin (TT)-binding gangliosides (Mirsky et al. 1978) in double-labeling experiments using immunofluorescence (Stallcup 1981) (Fig. 1). The results obtained depended on the age of the animal from which the cells were taken. When whole brain from 15-day embryos was dissociated and examined after 2 to 3 weeks in culture, approximately 10% of the cells that labeled with TT also labeled with anti-NG2. This accounted for approximately 50% of the anti-NG2-positive cells; the other 50% were negative for TT and were also negative for anti-GFAP and anti-GC. In 2- to 3-week-old cultures of cerebrum or cerebellum from older animals (19-day embryos to 4-day postnatal), some TT-positive cells were again seen to label with anti-NG2, but, in addition, 30–60% of NG2-positive cells also stained with anti-GFAP. GC-positive oligodendrocytes never labeled with anti-NG2.

At all ages, the NG2-positive cells had a characteristic morphology. Their cell bodies had diameters of about 10 μm and their processes were about 20–60 μm long, being shorter than typical mature neuronal processes. Double labeling with anti-GFAP and TT

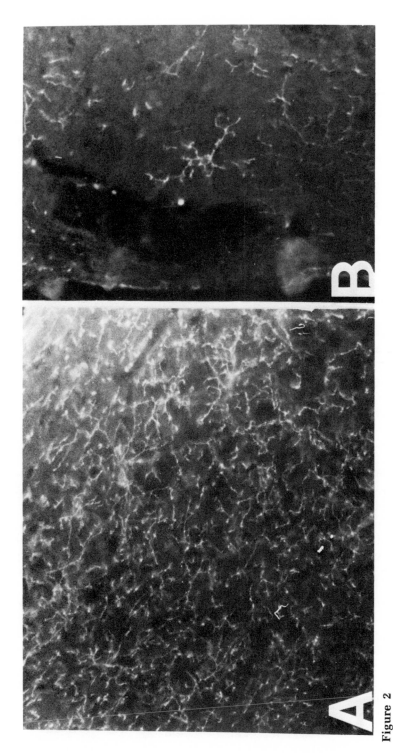

Figure 2

Staining with anti-NG2 in the adult rat pons. 15-μm frozen sections of the pons were cut from adult rats perfused with 0.1% glutaraldehyde and 1.0% paraformaldehyde. Sections were stained with rabbit anti-NG2, followed by fluorescein-labeled goat anti–rabbit IgG. (A) Most commonly seen are networks of fibers. (B) Occasionally a cell body with attached fibers is found.

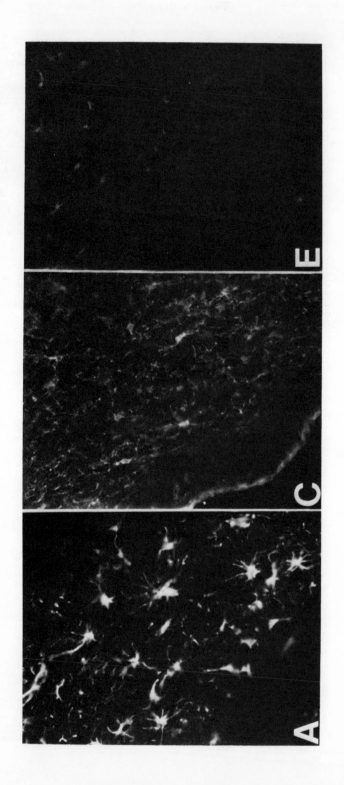

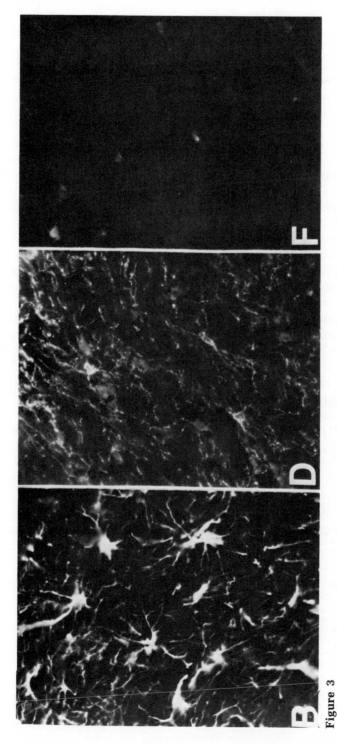

Figure 3

Staining with anti-GFAP and anti-NG2 in rat corpus callosum. 15-μm frozen sections were cut from adult rats perfused with 0.1% glutaraldehyde and 1.0% paraformaldehyde. Sections were stained with either rabbit anti-GFAP, rabbit anti-NG2, or, as a control, rabbit anti-NG2 absorbed with B49 cells, followed by fluorescein-labeled goat anti—rabbit IgG. (*A* and *B*) Anti-GFAP; (*C* and *D*) anti-NG2; (*E* and *F*) anti-NG2 absorbed with B49. Fields *A*, *C*, and *E* are magnified 352×. Fields *B*, *D*, and *F* are magnified 528×.

47

revealed that some cells were positive for both of these markers. Of these GFAP-positive, TT-positive cells, some had the characteristic morphology of NG2-positive cells, so it is likely that some cells are positive for all three markers.

These results show that there are interesting similarities between normal NG2-positive cells cultured from young animals and the seven cell lines that express NG2: In both cases the cells exhibit mixtures of neuronal and glial properties (Table 2).

As adult nervous tissue is not easy to culture, NG2 distribution was examined on cryostat sections of brain from adult rats perfused with 0.1% glutaraldehyde and 1% paraformaldehyde. Preliminary results show that there is staining with anti-NG2 (Fig. 2 shows examples of staining in the pons). In serial sections of corpus callosum, areas rich in GFAP-positive astrocytes also labeled with anti-NG2 (Fig. 3). Although definitive double-labeling experiments have not yet been done, some cells with similar morphologies are stained with both anti-GFAP and anti-NG2. However, NG2 cannot be a marker for all astrocytes since GFAP-positive radial glial fibers in the cerebellum were unlabeled with anti-NG2.

The conventional rabbit and mouse anti-NG2 precipitated a protein of approximately 300,000 daltons (by SDS-polyacrylamide gel electrophoresis) in preparations from all seven NG2-positive cell lines. When lines were cultured in the presence of radiolabeled sugars or amino acids, the 300,000-dalton band was radioactive, suggesting that NG2 is a glycoprotein.

To make an anti-NG2 reagent that was monospecific and would not need extensive adsorption, monoclonal antibodies were prepared. BALB/c mice were immunized with B49 cells, and their spleen cells were fused with the myeloma P3-X63-Ag (Köhler and Milstein 1975).

Table 2

Neuronal and Glial Properties of NG2$^+$ Cells

| | Primary cultures | | Cell lines | |
			pseudoneurons B82, B108, B19	pseudoglia B49, C6, B111, βHC
	early	late		
Neuronal properties	some TT binding	TT binding PC12 antigen	NA$^+$ channels K$^+$ channels N4 antigen	K$^+$ channels
Glial properties		G2 antigen GFAP	G2 antigen	G1 antigen (B49, C6, B111) G2 antigen (B49) GFAP (C6)

Supernatants from resultant clones were tested by RIA on B49 cells, and a monoclonal IgG1 was isolated (designated P11) that has the same properties as the conventional antisera with regard to the staining pattern of primary cultures.

In summary, NG2 is a cell-surface glycoprotein that is expressed on cells with some neuronal and some glial properties. NG2 may be a marker for stem cells capable of differentiating into either neurons or glia, or it may be a marker for a population of incompletely differentiated cells that are already committed to becoming either neurons or glia. Neither of these alternatives adequately explains the expression of NG2 on adult tissue, but preliminary evidence suggests that in the adult, NG2 is retained by a subpopulation of astrocytes.

REFERENCES

Arner, L. and W. Stallcup. 1981. Rubidium efflux from neural cell lines through voltage-dependent potassium channels. *Dev. Biol.* **83:**128.

Bignami, A., L. Eng, D. Dahl, and C. Uyeda. 1972. Localization of the glial fibrillary acidic protein in astrocytes by immunofluorescence. *Brain Res.* **43:**429.

Köhler, G. and C. Milstein. 1975. Continuous cultures of fused cells secreting antibody of predefined specificity. *Nature* **265:**495.

Mirsky, R., L. Wendon, P. Black, C. Stolkin, and D. Bray. 1978. Tetanus toxin: A cell surface marker for neurons in culture. *Brain Res.* **148:**251.

Raff, M., R. Mirsky, K. Fields, R. Lisak, S. Dorfman, D. Silberberg, N. Gregson, S. Leibowitz, and M. Kennedy. 1978. Galactocerebroside is a specific cell-surface antigenic marker for oligodendrocytes in culture. *Nature* **274:**813.

Schubert, D., S. Heinemann, W. Carlisle, H. Tarikas, B. Kimes, J. Patrick, J. Steinbach, W. Culp, and B. Brandt. 1974. Clonal cell lines from the rat central nervous system. *Nature* **249:**224.

Stallcup, W. 1981. The NG2 antigen, a putative lineage marker: Immunofluorescent localization in primary cultures of rat brain. *Dev. Biol.* **83:**147.

Stallcup, W. and M. Cohn. 1976. Correlation of surface antigens and cell type in cloned cell lines from the rat central nervous system. *Exp. Cell Res.* **98:**285.

Wilson, S., E. Baetge, and W. Stallcup. 1981. Antisera specific for cell lines with mixed neuronal and glial properties. *Dev. Biol.* **83:**139.

Monoclonal Antibodies and the Identification of Cerebellar Cell Lines

GREGORY GIOTTA

Developmental Biology Laboratory
The Salk Institute
San Diego, California 92138

• To study complex cell-cell interactions in the nervous system, it would be extremely useful to generate, in quantity, pure populations of characterized neural cells that exhibit a differentiated phenotype. A potentially powerful technique for doing this is described here. Normal neural cells were transformed with a temperature-sensitive (ts) RNA tumor virus to generate permanent cell lines from primary rat cerebellar cells (Giotta et al. 1980). The rationale for using ts Rous sarcoma virus (ts-RSV) is based on the work of others who have shown that cells infected with ts-RSV exhibit phenotypic alterations that appear to be under control of the ts transforming gene. This technique had been successfully applied previously to various cell types, including melanoblasts, erythroblasts, and myoblasts (Fiszman and Fuchs 1975; Holtzer et al. 1975; Boettiger et al. 1977; Graf et al. 1978; Fiszman 1978). At the permissive temperature, these cells exhibit a transformed phenotype and, similar to cells transformed by other techniques, display alterations in the differentiated properties characteristic of the cell type being studied. In contrast, at the nonpermissive temperature, cells transformed with ts-RSV assume a normal phenotype and express highly differentiated properties. To characterize the neural cell lines, monoclonal antibodies that recognize neural antigens were generated.

Normal cells were taken from neonatal rat cerebellum and infected with a strain of ts-RSV. Cells were grown at the permissive temperature for this virus (33–34°C) and were cloned to give stable cell lines. The temperature of the cultures was then raised to 38°C (the nonpermissive temperature for the virus) several days prior to

51

being assayed for the expression of differentiated properties. One cell line, WC5, clearly showed the potential of this technique. When WC5 is grown at the permissive temperature for the virus, it has a typical transformed morphology, but when kept at the nonpermissive temperature, the cells flatten out, and within four to seven days they express the astrocyte-specific antigen glial fibrillary acidic protein (GFAP), which is visualized by indirect immunofluorescence (Giotta and Cohn 1981).

To ascertain that this switch at the nonpermissive temperature was due to inactivation of the virus and not a direct effect of the temperature change, temperature-insensitive RSV variants were generated. By plating cells at a low density at the nonpermissive temperature for the virus, a few cells (~1 in 10,000) reverted to a transformed state after about ten days. This was indicated by (1) a transformed morphology, (2) lack of contact inhibition of growth, and (3) growth in agar at the permissive as well as the nonpermissive temperature, unlike the parent cells, which grow in agar only at the permissive temperature.

Several of these temperature-insensitive WC5 cell lines were not labeled by anti-GFAP regardless of whether they were grown at the permissive or nonpermissive temperature. This suggests that the ts virus suppresses GFAP expression in WC5 when this cell line is kept at the permissive temperature.

The results, though encouraging, were less clear cut for the neuronal lines. They expressed some, but not all, of the characteristics of differentiated neurons regardless of the time they are kept at the nonpermissive temperature. This is probably because successful transformation depends on cell division at the time of infection with virus, so that the viral genome can be integrated into the host genome. This means that only dividing, undifferentiated neuroblasts in early cerebellum can be successfully transformed. If it proves possible to make older, more differentiated neurons divide (e.g., with high K^+), more interesting cell lines may be generated.

After a number of cell lines had been generated from the cerebellum, the next step was to find out which cell type they represented in vivo. To do this, a range of monoclonal antibodies was produced that reacted with cerebellar cells. Spleen cells from BALB/c mice immunized with homogenates of rat cerebellum were fused with the mouse myeloma SP2/0-Ag14. The supernatants from resultant clones were tested on unfixed primary cerebellum cultures from 3-day-old rats, after the cultures were in vitro for several days. On the basis of this screening, monoclonal antibodies were grouped into several distinct categories according to whether the antigen they recognized was expressed on:

1. granule cells (both soma and neurites) (Figs. 1 and 2);

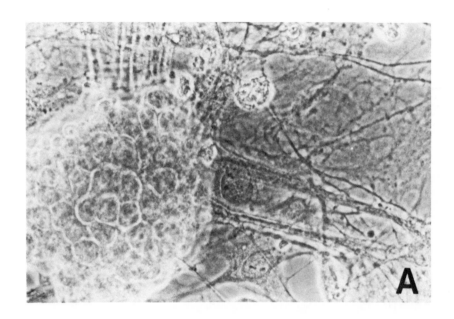

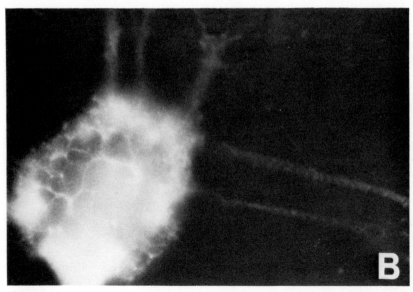

Figure 1
Staining of granule cell neurons in a cerebellar primary culture with a monoclonal antibody (C4/12) representative of group 1. The antibody labels both the cell soma and neurites of the granule neurons. Immunofluorescence staining was done by first incubating the cells with the monoclonal antibody, followed by subsequent washing and incubation with rhodamine-labeled goat anti−mouse IgG. Magnification, 800×.

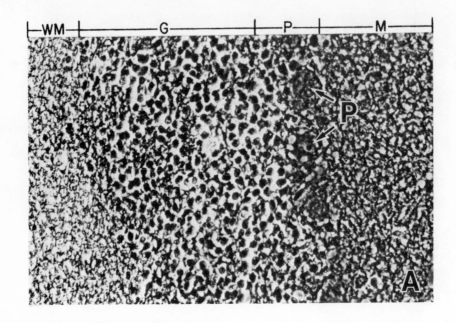

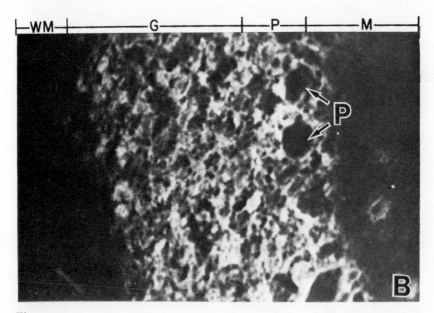

Figure 2
Staining of granule neurons in a frozen section of the cerebellum with C4/
12. Note that although the granule neuron cell bodies fluoresce, there is a
puzzling absence of fluorescence in the molecular layer that contains
granule neuron fibers. Magnification, 400×.

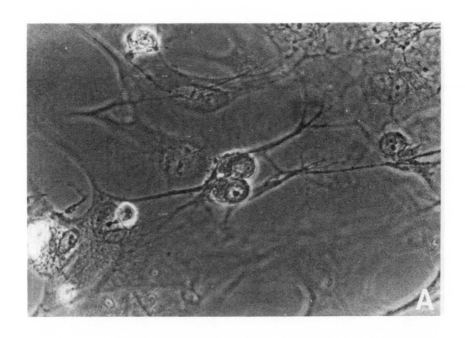

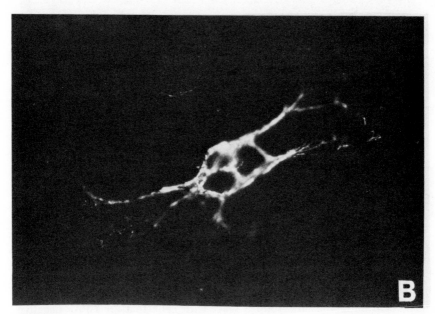

Figure 3
Staining of oligodendrocytes with a group-2 monoclonal antibody. Magnification, 800×.

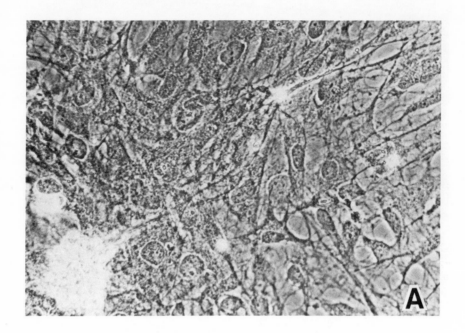

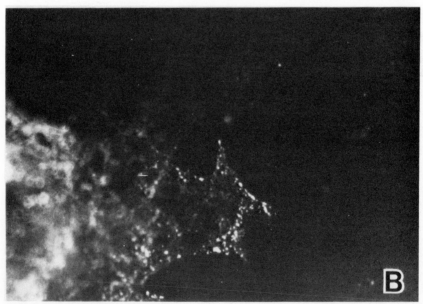

Figure 4
Monoclonal antibodies in group 5 react with cells that are GFAP-negative and have an epithelioid morphology. Often these cells are found beneath bundles of granule neurons. Magnification, 400×.

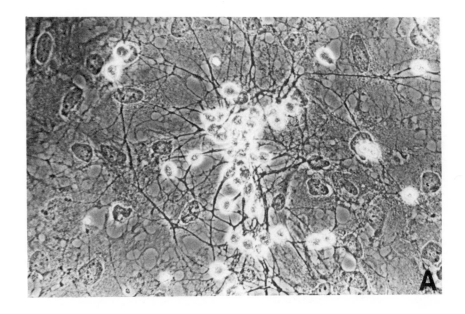

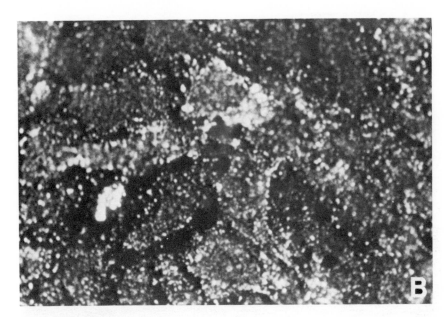

Figure 5
An example of the cell types that react with a group-4 monoclonal antibody.
Note that the antibody reacts primarily with "flat" cells and not granule cell
neurons. Magnification, 400×.

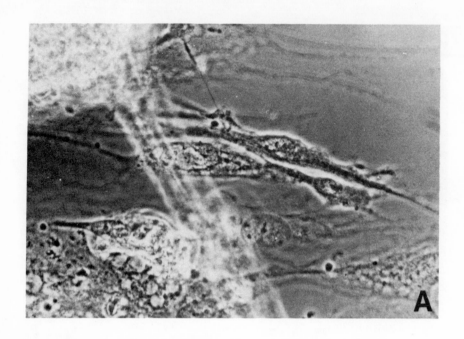

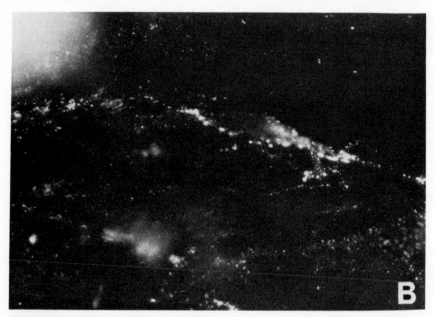

Figure 6
Group-5 monoclonal antibodies react with all cell types. Magnification, 400×.

2. oligodendrocytes (the staining pattern resembles those of the O antigens; see Schachner et al., this volume) (Fig. 3);
3. islands of flat cells with epithelioid morphology (probably not astrocytes) (Fig. 4);
4. all flat cells (Fig. 5);
5. all cell types (Fig. 6).

The ts-RSV-derived cell lines that had been generated from cerebellar cells were screened for binding of these monoclonal antibodies. None of the lines expressed antigens recognized by group-2 antibodies, either at the permissive or the nonpermissive temperature. All cell lines expressed one or more of the antigens recognized in groups 1, 3, 4, and 5. All but one of the cell lines, regardless of their glial or neuronal nature, expressed the group-1 antigen, which marks only granule cells in culture (this antibody is designated C4/12). One cell line expressed C4/12 binding at the permissive temperature but not at the nonpermissive temperature, perhaps suggesting that this cell line arose from a cell that in vivo was a precursor cell destined to lose this antigen in development. Some of the cell lines that stained with group-3 antibodies also lost the antigen at the nonpermissive temperature.

In summary, we have generated a number of hybridomas that produce monoclonal antibodies specific for different types of cerebellar cells. We are using these antibodies to establish the nature of cell lines derived from the cerebellum with the aim of developing an in vitro model system to study cerebellar development.

ACKNOWLEDGMENT

We thank the March of Dimes for supporting this work (grant no. 5-229).

REFERENCES

Boettiger, D., K. Roby, J. Brumbaugh, J. Biehl, and H. Holtzer. 1977. Transformation of chicken embryo retinal melanoblasts by a temperature-sensitive mutant of Rous sarcoma virus. Cell 11:811.

Fiszman, M. Y. and P. Fuchs. 1975. Temperature sensitive expression of differentiation in transformed myoblasts. Nature 254:429.

Giotta, G. J. and M. Cohn. 1981. Expression of glial fibrillary acidic protein in a rat cerebellar cell line. J. Cell. Physiol. 107:219.

Giotta, G. J., J. Heitzmann, and M. Cohn. 1980. Properties of two temperature-sensitive Rous sarcoma virus transformed cerebellar cell lines. Brain Res. 202:445.

Graf, T., N. Ade, and H. Beug. 1978. Temperature-sensitive mutant of erythroblastosis virus suggests a block of differentiation as a mechanism of leukaemogenesis. *Nature* **275:**496.

Holtzer, H., J. Biehl, G. Yeoh, and A. Kaji. 1975. Effect of oncogenic virus on muscle differentiation. *Proc. Natl. Acad. Sci.* **72:**4051.

Monoclonal Antibodies That Define Neural Cell-surface Molecules in the Mammalian Central and Peripheral Nervous Systems

JAMES COHEN, RHONA MIRSKY, STEPHANIE RATTRAY, SIVAYOGI SELVENDREN, and TOM VULLIAMY

Neuroimmunology Group
Department of Zoology
University College London
London, England WCIE 6BT

• For the past few years, tetanus toxin (TT), which binds to long-chain gangliosides on neurons, has been utilized as a cell-surface marker for cultured vertebrate neurons (Dimpfel et al. 1977; Mirsky et al. 1979; Mirsky 1980). The cell adhesion molecule (CAM), a glycoprotein found in chick (Rutishauser et al. 1978), and the closely related D2 antigen in rat (Jorgenson and Moller 1980) seem to have a similar distribution to that of TT receptors. More recently, a monoclonal antibody to a cell-surface ganglioside (GQ) has been described with similar specificity (Eisenbarth et al. 1979, but see Eisenbarth et al., this volume). In addition, a number of intracellular, neuron-specific antigens have been described, such as 14-3-2 (neuronal enolase) (Schmechel et al. 1978) and the neurofilament antigens, and certain subpopulations of neurons can be distinguished according to the transmitters they make, either by catecholamine-induced fluorescence or by antibodies to the transmitters or transmitter-synthesizing enzymes. However, so far, antibodies that can distinguish subpopulations of neurons on the basis of cell-surface differences have not been described. Since antibodies to surface antigens bind to living cells, they have the added advantage of providing a means of specifically eliminating or purifying the antigen-bearing cells from mixed cell populations.

The hybridoma technique (Köhler and Milstein 1975) was used to produce two monoclonal antibodies that recognize neural cell-surface antigens. Interestingly, one of them (A4) reacts only with neurons that have their cell bodies in the central nervous system (CNS), whereas

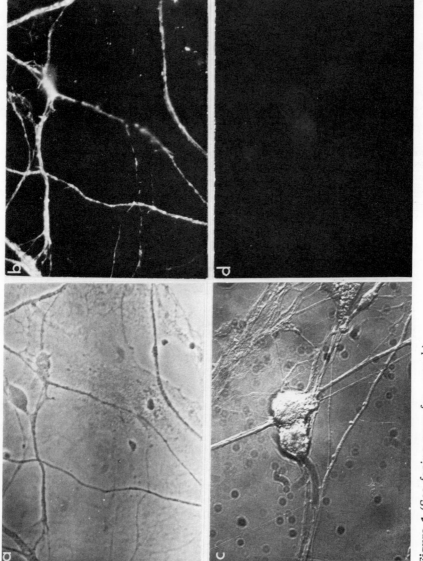

Figure 1 (See facing page for legend.)

the other (38/D7) reacts only with neurons that have their cell bodies in the peripheral nervous system (PNS).

A4 was produced by immunizing mice with dissociated cultures of rat cerebellum, whereas 38/D7 was produced by immunizing mice with dissociated cell cultures of neonatal rat dorsal root ganglia (DRG). In both cases, the cultures were treated with cytosine arabinoside to enrich for neurons. Living cells were scraped off the culture dishes and injected into BALB/c mice whose spleen cells were fused with NS1 (P3-NS1/1Ag4-1) myeloma cells.

CLONE A4

• A4 (Cohen and Selvendren 1981) produces an IgM monoclonal antibody that in indirect fluorescence assays binds to all TT-positive neurons in a variety of rat CNS cultures, including cerebrum, cerebellum, hippocampus, retina, and olfactory bulb, but does not bind to neurons in DRG, superior cervical ganglion (SCG), or nodose ganglion cultures (Fig. 1). It binds to no other cell type tested except a subpopulation of astrocytes in optic nerve cultures, a distribution also exhibited by TT receptors.

The distribution of antigen in vivo was examined by indirect immunofluorescence in cryostat sections (6 μm) of immature cerebellum (postnatal day 16). Sections were double-labeled with both antibody A4 (Fig. 2 c and f) and rabbit anti–glial fibrillary acidic protein (anti-GFAP) (Fig. 2 b and e), an intracellular glia-specific marker, so as to contrast the pattern of radial glial staining with the neuronal specificity of antibody A4 binding. With A4, ring fluorescence was clearly seen around the majority of cell bodies in the external granular layer (Fig. 2c) and with lower intensity around the large Purkinje perikarya and small cells in the internal granular layer (Fig. 2f). No intracellular staining was seen with A4, and white matter (not shown) was only weakly positive. A quantitative absorption assay was used to detect the antigen recognized by A4 in homogenates of

Figure 1
A4 binding to rat CNS, but not to PNS, neurons. Cells in cultures of 6-day-old rat cerebella (a,b) or DRG (c,d) were labeled after 5 days in culture with antibody A4 (1:100 dilution of immune ascites from a mouse carrying a peritoneal A4-hybridoma tumor), followed by rhodamine-conjugated goat anti–mouse immunoglobulin (Cappel Ltd.; 1:100), fixed in acetic acid:ethanol (5:95), and then viewed with phase contrast (a) or Nomarski (c) and fluorescence (b,d) optics. Note that cerebellar neurons and their processes, but not the underlying fibroblastic cells, are labeled in b, whereas the prominent sensory neurons in d are A4-negative.

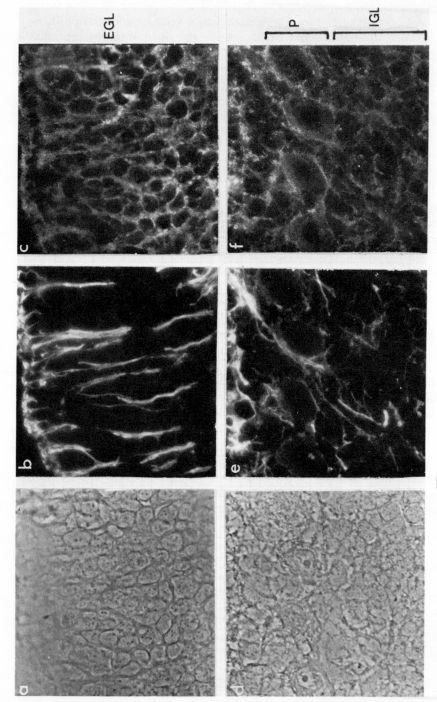

Figure 2 *(See facing page for legend.)*

64

developing brain. The antigen is not detectable in the 8-day embryo but is seen at a low level in the 10-day embryo. By the time of birth, the concentration in brain increases 30-fold per unit wet weight. At birth, the cerebellum (which develops postnatally in rodents) has only 3% of the maximal adult level; the adult level is attained by three weeks of age.

The antigen is expressed by all mammals tested except mouse and guinea pig. It is not detectable in frog or chick nervous tissue. The molecule is trypsin-, pronase-, and neuraminidase-resistant but is destroyed by boiling.

CLONE 38/D7

• Clone 38/D7 (Vulliamy et al. 1981) produces an IgM monoclonal antibody that in indirect immunofluorescence assays binds to TT-positive neurons in cultured rat DRG, SCG, and nodose ganglion but not to any of the neurons in cultured CNS that are positive for A4.

38/D7 binds to primary cultures of adrenal medulla that have been maintained in nerve growth factor (NGF); double staining for noradrenaline (NA) and 38/D7 shows that the 38/D7 binds to the NA-producing chromaffin cells of the adrenal medulla. The pheochromo-cytoma PC12 is also weakly positive for 38/D7. All other normal cells and cell lines tested are unlabeled by 38/D7. The antibody shows rather weak staining in cultured cells by indirect immunofluores-cence, and the more-sensitive immunoperoxidase technique was used to visualize staining of neurons in cryostat sections of DRG from adult rats perfused with 4% formaldehyde. The low levels of 38/D7 antibody binding have so far precluded the use of quantitative assays.

To examine the expression of the 38/D7 antigen in development, embryonic DRG cultures were double-stained with 38/D7 and TT. Although TT-positive neurons in 24-hour cultures of 14-day embry-onic DRG cultures were 38/D7-negative, by 48 hours they were 38/D7-positive; neurons in 15-day embryonic DRG cultures were 38/D7-positive when first studied at 24 hours (Fig. 3).

Figure 2

Localization of A4 binding in adolescent (P16) cerebellum. Small blocks of freshly dissected cerebellum were frozen in isopentane. Sections (6 μm) were cut on a cryostat at $-15°C$ and then incubated simultaneously with antibody A4 (supernatant 14) and rabbit anti-GFAP (1:200). After washing, binding was visualized by incubating with goat anti−rabbit immunoglobulin fluores-cein (1:100), and rhodamine-conjugated sheep anti−mouse immunoglobulin (1:100) sections were viewed by phase (a,d) or fluorescence (b,c,e,f) optics. (b,e) GFAP; (c,f) A4; (EGL) external granular layer; (P) Purkinje layer; (IGL) internal granular layer.

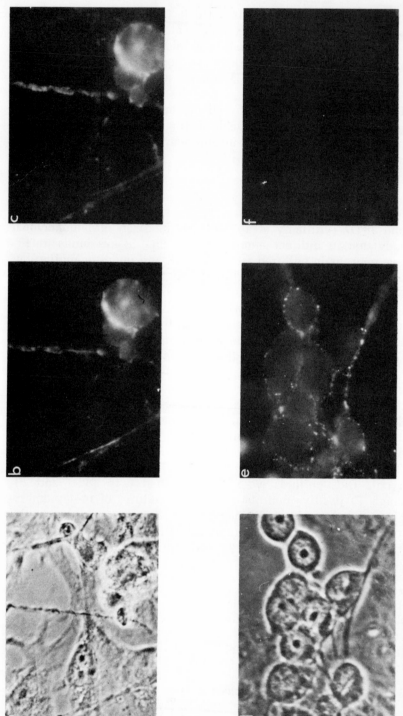

66

Figure 3 (See facing page for legend.)

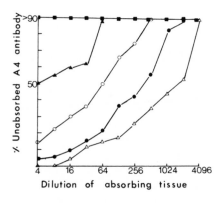

Figure 4
Quantitative absorption analysis of A4-immune ascites with rat CNS tissues of various ages. A4-immune ascites (50 μl; 1:250) were added to 50 μl portions of doubling dilutions of 50% (v/v) tissue homogenates in MEM-HEPES and incubated for 45 min on ice. After centrifugation, the residual antibody A4 in aliquots (50 μl) of supernatant was assayed for binding to microwell cultures of 6-day-old rat cerebella using ^{125}I-labeled rabbit anti—mouse μ heavy-chain immunoglobulin (50–100,000 cpm/well) as second antibody. The washed microtiter plates were cut up and individual wells assayed for bound radioactivity in a gamma counter. (*Ordinate*) Residual antibody A4 expressed as a percentage of the maximal binding obtained with unabsorbed immune ascites (1:500). (■) 8-day whole embryo; (▲) 10-day embryo brain; (○) newborn cerebellum; (●) 7-day-old cerebellum; (Δ) adult cerebellum.

Figure 3
38/D7 labeling of mature, but not embryonic, neurons. (a) Phase contrast micrograph of a DRG culture from a 5- to 6-day-old rat. Neuronal cell body is above the plane of nonneuronal cells and slightly out of focus. (b) TT and (c) 38/D7 labeling of the same cell, visualized by double-label indirect immunofluorescence. Nonneuronal cells are not labeled. (d) Phase contrast micrograph of neurons in DRG culture from 13-day embryonic rat after 48 hours in vitro. (e) TT labels, but (f) 38/D7 does not label, these neurons. Double immunofluorescent staining: Cells on collagen-coated coverslips were incubated with 3–5 μg/ml TT diluted in minimum essential medium (MEM)-HEPES with 5% fetal calf serum (FCS) for 30 min at room temperature. After washing with MEM-HEPES, rabbit anti—TT together with 38/D7 antibodies were added in 40 μl volumes for 30 min at room temperature. Bound immunoglobulin was detected by a further incubation for 30 min with fluorescein-conjugated goat anti—rabbit immunoglobulin (Nordic Ltd.; diluted 1:50 in MEM-HEPES plus 5% FCS) together with tetramethyl rhodamine-conjugated goat anti—mouse immunoglobulin (Cappell Ltd.; diluted 1:100). The cells were then fixed in 5% acetic acid in ethanol for 20 min at −20°C, mounted in glycerol with phenylenediamine, and sealed with nail varnish.

The 38/D7 antigen is restricted to rat. It is trypsin-sensitive, suggesting that it is a protein.

In summary, two monoclonal antibodies have been produced that distinguish central (A4) from peripheral (38/D7) neurons. They therefore recognize neurons of different embryological origins — CNS neurons originate in the neural tube in embryogenesis, whereas PNS neurons (and chromaffin cells) are derived from the neural crest or placodes. As such, these antibodies represent valuable, new cell-surface markers for neurons. Furthermore, they should provide an efficient means of purifying antigen-bearing cells with a view to establishing homogeneous cultures of neurons from the CNS or PNS in which the requirement for survival and growth may be studied in the absence of other cell types. Further work is needed to characterize the antigens and to reveal what their functions might be. Attempts to perturb neuronal function and growth with the monoclonal antibodies might yield important clues.

REFERENCES

Cohen, J. and S. Selvendren. 1981. Antibody against neuronal cell-surface antigen specific for CNS neurones. Nature (in press).

Dimpfel, W., R.T.C. Huang, and E. Habermann. 1977. Gangliosides in nervous tissue cultures and binding of ^{125}I-labelled tetanus toxin, a neuronal marker. J. Neurochem. 29:329.

Eisenbarth, G.S., F.S. Walsh, and M. Nirenberg. 1979. Monoclonal antibody to a plasma membrane antigen of neurones. Proc. Natl. Acad. Sci. 76:4913.

Jorgensen, O.S. and M. Moller. 1980. Immunocytochemical demonstration of the D2 protein in the presynaptic complex. Brain Res. 194:419.

Köhler, G. and C. Milstein. 1975. Continuous cultures of fused cells secreting antibody of predefined specificity. Nature 256:495.

Mirsky, R. 1980. Cell type-specific markers in nervous system cultures. Trends Neurosci. 4:190.

Mirsky, R., L.M.B. Wendon, P. Black, C. Stolkin, and D. Bray. 1978. Tetanus toxin—A cell surface marker for neurones in culture. Brain Res. 148:251.

Rutishauser, U., J.P. Thiery, R. Brackenburg, and G.M. Edelman. 1978. Adhesion among neural cells of the chick embryo. III. Relationship of the surface molecule CAM to cell adhesion and the development of histotypic patterns. J. Cell Biol. 79:371.

Schmechel, D., P.J. Marangos, M. Brightman, and F.K. Goodwin. 1978. Brain enolases as specific markers of neuronal and glial cells. Science 199:313.

Vulliamy, T., S. Rattray, and R. Mirsky. 1981. Sensory and autonomic peripheral neurones express a cell surface antigen not expressed by central neurones. Nature (in press).

Expression of the Major Histocompatibility Antigens in the Human Nervous System

LOIS A. LAMPSON

Department of Anatomy, School of Medicine
University of Pennsylvania
Philadelphia, Pennsylvania 19104

• The gene products of the major histocompatibility complex (MHC) are known to play an important role in recognition and mediation of cellular interactions in the immune system. The two major types of human MHC gene products are the class-I molecules (HLA-A, -B, and -C), which are thought to be expressed on all human nucleated cells, and class-II molecules (Ia-like), which have a restricted tissue distribution.

In the study reported here, monoclonal antibodies were used to determine the distribution of these antigens in the human nervous system.

Class-I molecules consist of two protein subunits: an HLA chain (m.w. ~43,000) that bears the polymorphic determinants expressed by these molecules, and an invariant β_2-microglobulin chain (m.w. 12,000). Two monoclonal antibodies were used to detect class-I molecules: W6/32 (Barnstable et al. 1978), which recognizes a nonpolymorphic determinant on the HLA chain, and L368, which is specific for β_2-microglobulin (L.A. Lampson et al., in prep.) (Fig. 1, left). To detect class-II molecules, L203 and L227 antibodies were used, which recognize nonpolymorphic determinants on two forms of these molecules (Lampson and Levy 1980) (Fig. 1, right). Various cell lines and tissue homogenates were tested. All were lightly fixed with 0.1% glutaraldehyde at room temperature. Cells and tissue homogenates were studied by radioimmunoassay, both in direct-binding assays and in more-sensitive competitive-binding assays (L. A. Lampson et al., in prep.). The results shown in Table 1 demonstrate that class-II molecules are not present on neural tissue (Koyoma et al. 1977), whereas

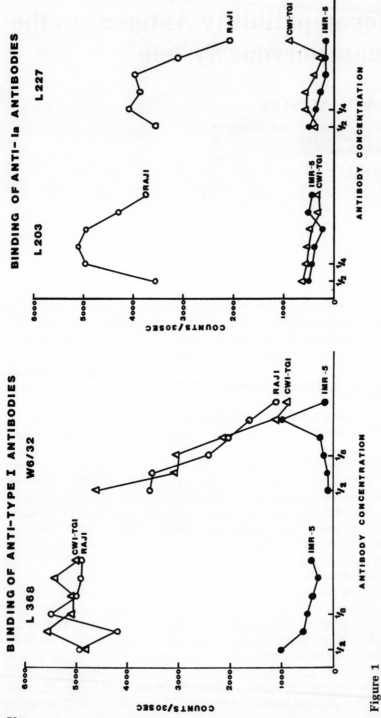

Figure 1

Direct binding of monoclonal antibodies to human cell lines. Raji is a B-cell line, CW1-TG1 is derived from an oligodendroglioma, and IMR-5 is derived from neuroblastoma. Culture medium containing the myeloma protein MOPC-21 was used as a negative control and gave binding values of a few hundred counts per 30 sec against the different cell lines.

Table 1
Expression of MHC Antigens by Human Neural Tissue

	Class-I antigen	Class-II antigen
Cell lines		
T lymphoblastoid	++	0
B lymphoblastoid	++	++
Oligodendroglioma (CW1-TG1-3865)	++	0
Neuroblastomas		
(IMR-5, NMB, CHP-134, SK-N-SH)	±	0
Normal tissue		
Spleen	++	+
Brain	+	0

class-I molecules are present on neural tissue (Nilsson et al. 1973; Welsh et al. 1977).

REFERENCES

Barnstable, C.J., W.F. Bodmer, G. Brown, G. Galfre, C. Milstein, A.F. Williams, and A. Ziegler. 1978. Production of monoclonal antibodies to group A erythrocytes, HLA and other human cell surface antigens—New tools for genetic analysis. *Cell* **14**:9.

Koyoma, K., K. Nakamuro, N. Tanigaki, and D. Pressman. 1977. Alloantigens of human lymphoid cell lines; "human Ia-like antigens." *Immunology* **33**:217.

Lampson, L.A. and R. Levy. 1980. Two populations of Ia-like molecules on a human B cell line. *J. Immunol.* **125**:293.

Nilsson, K., P.E. Evrin, I. Berggard, and J. Ponten. 1973. Involvement of lymphoid and nonlymphoid cells in the production of β_2-microglobulin—A homologue of the constant domains of IgG. *Nat. New Biol.* **244**:44.

Welsh, K.I., G. Dorval, and K. Nilsson. 1977. Quantitation of β_2-microglobulin and HLA on the surface of human cells. *Scand. J. Immunol.* **6**:265.

Immunochemical Studies of Avian Peripheral Neurogenesis

GARY CIMENT and JAMES A. WESTON

Department of Biology
University of Oregon
Eugene, Oregon 97403

• Cells of the sensory ganglia of vertebrates contain at least two neuronal types as well as glial elements, all of which are derived from the neural crest (NC). We wish to establish at what time during development and under what environmental conditions the cell lineages leading to these various cell types get established. To do so we need good operational markers for the various neuronal cell types. To this end, monoclonal antibodies have been produced for cytochemical staining that may be applied (1) to identify and characterize lineage-specific antigens, (2) to discover whether these antigens play a role in subsequent developmental events (e.g., as receptors for cellular interactions), and (3) to determine the temporal order of restrictions that could define the overall pattern of lineages in NC-cell development.

The NC is a structure that exists only transiently following neurulation in the early embryo. After an extensive migration, NC cells differentiate into diverse cell types, including pigment, endocrine, paracrine, skeletal, as well as peripheral and central nervous system elements (Weston 1970). It is widely asserted that the cells of the NC are "pluripotent," in the sense that in response to environmental stimuli encountered during migration or after localization, all cells of this population are able to give rise to any of the phenotypes of the crest repertoire (Le Douarin et al. 1977). This belief is based on heterotopic transplantation in vivo of crest-cell populations by Noden (1978a,b) and Le Douarin and coworkers (Le Douarin et al. 1978; Le Douarin 1980), who found that undifferentiated and partially differentiated NC cells differentiated according to their location rather than their source when transplanted into a new tissue environment.

73

Likewise, cells of NC-derived tissues also respond to environmental conditions in vitro so that new crest phenotypes appear adventitiously (Patterson and Chun 1974; Nichols and Weston 1977). In some experiments, such metaplasia has been shown to occur in a single cell (Patterson 1978; Loring et al. 1979), which eliminates the possibility that altered phenotypes result from the selection of subpopulations within an initially heterogeneous cell mixture.

It is possible that initially homogeneous populations of NC cells segregate developmental lineages analogous to those described in simpler systems (see, e.g., Kauffman et al. 1978; Tomozawa and Sueoka 1978). This notion of developmental lineages suggests that some NC-derived cell types may be more closely related phenotypically than other derivatives of the NC. In addition, developmental restrictions would be expected to occur in a specific order as the NC cells encounter a sequence of environmental cues during their morphogenetic phase. There is, as yet, no direct evidence that cell lineages in NC development exist (Weston 1981).

Surface antigenic determinants on differentiating sensory neurons allow the following developmental questions to be asked:

1. At a particular developmental age, is the expression of an antigen confined exclusively to a particular cell type (i.e., sensory neurons)? If so, is it also found on other developmentally closely related types (e.g., sympathetic neurons)? Or, by analogy to the Thy-1 antigen (Fields 1979), is it found on diverse cell types only distantly related (e.g., cells derived from the other germ layers)?

2. In a particular cell's development, at what stage does the antigenic determinant appear, and does it disappear at later stages? Is the antigen present on undifferentiated NC cells? If so, is it found on all of the cells or on a few? Can the antigen's presence be used to identify premigratory NC cells? If the antigen later disappears during sensory neurogenesis, is it retained by other NC-derived cell types? The answers to these questions would address the theoretical notion of developmental lineages during NC differentiation leading to a particular crest derivative and would suggest where restrictive events might occur at intermediate stages in development.

3. Are all sensory neurons equivalent with respect to the presence of a particular antigen? If not, are the differences related to cell lineage or developmental stage, or do differences in antigen distribution underlie some other important functional differences in the cells that have yet to be discovered (such as neurotransmitter uptake mechanisms)?

4. What are the molecular properties of the antigen?

5. What is the function of the antigen? Is the function related to a basic developmental process (such as a receptor for inductive cellular interactions), or is the antigen related to the phenotype of the cell (e.g., voltage-dependent channels might be recognized as antigens on neuronal cell surfaces)?

METHODS

• Hybridoma cell lines were produced by the polyethylene-glycol-induced fusion of SP2/0 cells (Shulman et al. 1978) with splenocytes obtained from a mouse immunized three times with 7-day embryonic chick sensory ganglia. This particular ganglionic age was chosen because it provided a wide range of neuronal developmental stages— from premitotic neuroblasts to fully differentiated, functioning neurons (Hamburger and Levi-Montalcini 1949). The resultant hybridoma cell lines were screened for production of monoclonal antibodies using an indirect immunoperoxidase-staining method. Positive cell lines were then cloned by limited-dilution methods (1 cell per well— verified by visual inspection) and rescreened.

Briefly, the screening method involved placing conditioned medium from each of 128 growth-positive hybridoma wells into separate wells of 96-well plates containing paraformaldehyde-fixed cultures of 9-day-old chick sensory ganglia (trypsin-dissociated and cultured for 5 days prior to fixation). Following an overnight incubation at 4°C, the medium was removed, the cell layer washed extensively with buffer, and then the following reagents were added in successive 1-hour periods, followed by extensive buffer washes: (1) rabbit anti—mouse IgG, IgA, and IgM; (2) goat anti—rabbit IgG; and (3) peroxidase/rabbit antiperoxidase. The presence of peroxidase activity on the cell surface (indicative of MC antibodies binding to the cells) was visualized using the Hanker-Yates reagent (Hanker et al. 1977). The 96 wells were then filled with glycerin jelly and sealed for optical clarity.

This method of screening has several advantages over those methods utilizing ^{125}I-labeled immunoreagents: (1) It allows us to use many fewer target cells per well (50 cells per well is more than sufficient); (2) it allows us to use a mixed population of morphologically distinguishable cells (i.e., round, phase-bright neurons vs flat, phase-gray nonneuronal cells) as intrinsic specificity controls; and (3) the same methodology can be readily adapted for ultrastructural studies since the enzymatic products of the peroxidase reaction are insoluble and electron-dense.

In more recent experiments, horseradish peroxidase was directly conjugated to one of the antibodies (E/C8) using the periodate technique of Nakane and Kawaoi (1974). For immunocytochemical stains, these peroxidase-conjugated antibodies were incubated with paraformaldehyde-fixed cells, the cells were then washed extensively with buffer, and then peroxidase activity was visualized as above. This direct immunoperoxidase staining method has several advantages over the indirect stain, including (1) decreasing the amount of time and the number of reagents used, (2) allowing a more-quantitative estimate of the density of antigenic sites (since the number of peroxidase molecules is related to the number of antigenic determinants in a stoichiometric fashion), and (3) permitting binding-competition studies to be performed, which can be used to determine whether two antibodies bind to a common determinant.

RESULTS

Qualitatively Different Classes of Monoclonal Antibodies

• Twelve clones of hybridoma cells have been isolated that make antibodies against subpopulations of cultured sensory ganglionic cells. We have assigned the antibodies to three qualitatively distinct classes on the basis of their staining patterns:

1. One class of antibody (Table 1) stains the cell bodies of a subpopulation of neurons. The staining is usually uniform (see Figs. 1 and 2) but occasionally seems to be localized to one side of the soma. The overall proportion of antigen-positive neurons varies from 10% to 30% of the total number of identifiable neurons. The neurites of these cells are unstained, even when large excesses of the antibody are added. Cells that are typically nonneuronal in morphology (i.e., phase-gray, flattened) do not stain. In some cultures, rare antigen-positive cells have been observed that do not have an obvious neuronal morphology. Whether these anomalous cells are immature postmitotic neurons (see Chalozonitis and Fischbach 1980), neuroblasts, or some other cell type, remains to be determined.

2. Monoclonal antibodies of the second class (Table 1) stain fibers as well as somas of a subpopulation of neurons (again, the proportion is a variable 10–30%). The staining is occasionally patchy, but uniformly stained neurons can also be seen (Fig. 3). One curious feature in the staining pattern of antibodies of this class is the presence of intermittent dense staining along the neurites (see Fig. 4). These antigen-positive regions are seldom longer than 100 μm and frequently appear in chains. At present, we think that these regions may be either (1) axon-substratum attachment sites, (2) varicosities of

Table 1
Cellular Localization of Staining with Various Monoclonal Antibodies, Using Various Cultured Cell Types as Target Cells

Antibody-producing hybridoma clones	neuronal somata[1]	Sensory ganglion cells			Somitic mesenchymal cells	Heart fibroblasts
		fibers	flattened, non-neuronal cells	anomalous cells[2]		
A/C8	+, sub[3]	0	0	+	0	0
E/A6	+, sub	0	0	+	0	0
E/B4	+, sub	0	0	+	0	0
A/C6	+, sub	+	0	0	0	0
A/D10	+, sub	+	0	0	0	0
E/C4	+, sub	+	0	0	0	0
E/C8	+, sub	+	0	0	0	0
E/E1	+, sub	+	0	0	0	0
E/E7	+, sub	+	0	0	0	0
C/B2	variable	0	+	+	+	+
E/F4	variable	0	+	+	not done	not done
-/C9	variable	0	+	+	+	+

[1] Neuronal somata are defined as large, round, phase-bright cells with processes.
[2] Anomalous cells are not neuronal (by the above criteria) but are spindle-shaped and associated with neuronal aggregates, rather than flattened and phase-gray like glial and fibroblastic cells. These cells may be postmitotic neuroblasts, as described by Chalozinitis and Fishbach (1980).
[3] Subpopulations of cells stained.

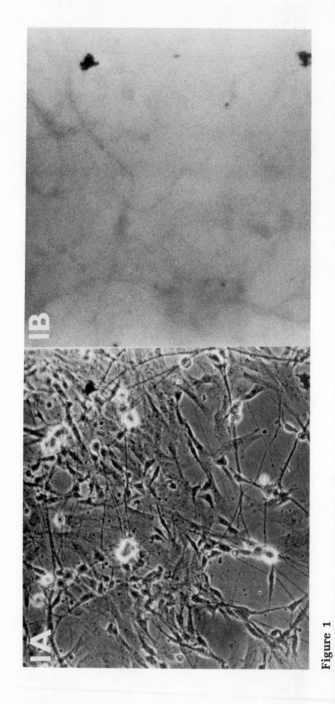

Figure 1
Negative control of the indirect immunoperoxidase-staining method. The cells are from trypsin-dissociated, 9-day embryonic chick sensory ganglia cultured for 5 days and then fixed in paraformaldehyde (2.5%). (*A*) Phase contrast; (*B*) bright-field illumination of cells in A. (Use the debris for registration of the images.)

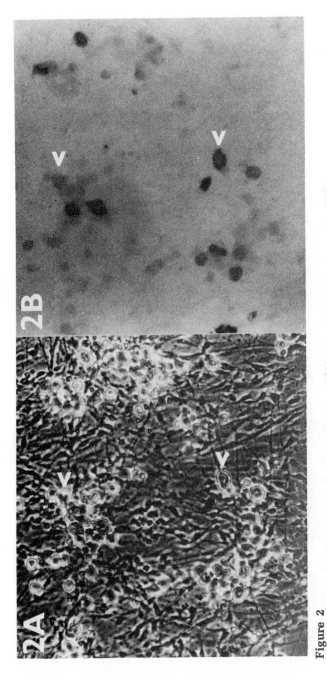

Figure 2
Staining of sensory ganglion cells by E/B4 monoclonal antibody, as described in the legend to Fig. 1. (A) Phase contrast; (B) bright-field illumination of cells in A. The upper arrows in A and B point to a neuron that is only marginally stained; the lower arrows point to a neuron that is heavily stained.

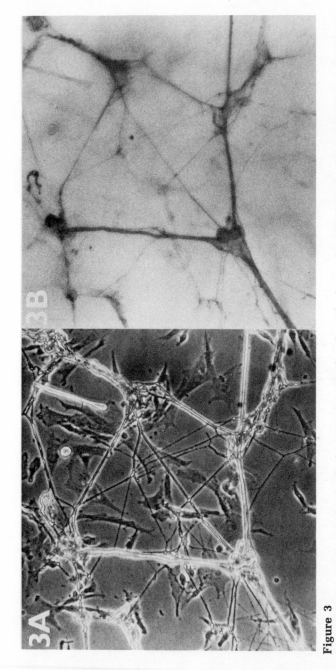

Figure 3
Staining of sensory ganglion cells by A/D10 monoclonal antibody, as described in the legend to Fig. 1. (A) Phase contrast; (B) bright-field illumination of cells in A.

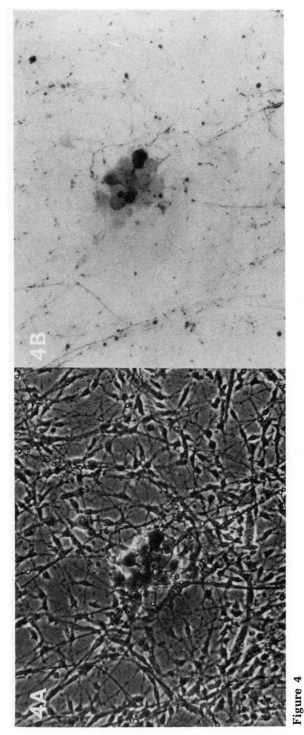

Figure 4

Staining of 8-day embryonic quail sensory ganglia by E/C8 monoclonal antibody (trypsin-dissociated and cultured 5 days prior to paraformaldehyde fixation). (A) Phase contrast; (B) bright-field illumination of cells in A.

some sort, or possibly (3) structures analogous to those described by Nuttall and Wessells (1979) in ciliary ganglionic
neurons. In any case, we will be looking at these regions in
more detail using transmission electron microscopy.
3. The third class of antibody (Table 1) binds at high concentration to nearly all cell types in sensory ganglia, but only to
nonneuronal cells at lower concentrations. This variability in
the pattern of staining may be the result of quantitative differences in the density of an antigenic determinant common to
both neuronal and nonneuronal cells in the ganglion.

The three general patterns of binding among the 12 monoclonal
antibodies indicate that there are at least three different antigenic
determinants being recognized by the various antibodies. However,
additional preliminary evidence using peroxidase-conjugated E/C8
antibody (E/C8-HRP) suggests that the minimum number of determinants is at least four. In this study, the subsequent binding of E/C8-
HRP was blocked only by prior treatment of ganglion cultures with
A/C6. Other monoclonal antibodies within this class (see 2 in list
above) presumably bind at other sites.

Cellular Specificity of Monoclonal Antibody Binding

In addition to the internal specificity controls inherent in the mixed
cultures of chick sensory ganglia used to screen the hybridoma supernatants, we have also screened other cultured cell types as targets for
binding (Table 1). In these studies, quail sensory ganglia from 8-day
embryos (roughly equivalent in maturity to 9-day chick embryos)
were found to bind the antibodies in an identical pattern to that of
chick (e.g., Fig. 4 and Table 1). In contrast, quail mesodermal derivatives such as somitic mesenchyme (Fig. 5) and heart fibroblasts (not
shown) only bound one antibody (G/C9) of the third, less-specific
category.

Of particular interest is the binding pattern to apparently undifferentiated quail neural crest cells, which are thought to be the direct
antecedents of sensory neurons (Weston 1970). With some of the
monoclonal antibodies (e.g., E/C8), only a subpopulation of these cells
stained. Moreover, many of the antigen-positive cells had a striking
neuronlike morphology, sending out long, neuritelike fibers (see Fig.
6). In contrast, other antibodies stained all of the crest cells (e.g.,
E/A6; not shown) and typically in a patchy fashion. It has yet to be
determined whether these antigens are present on NC cells at such
early ages in vivo or whether these antigens are expressed preco-
ciously in culture.

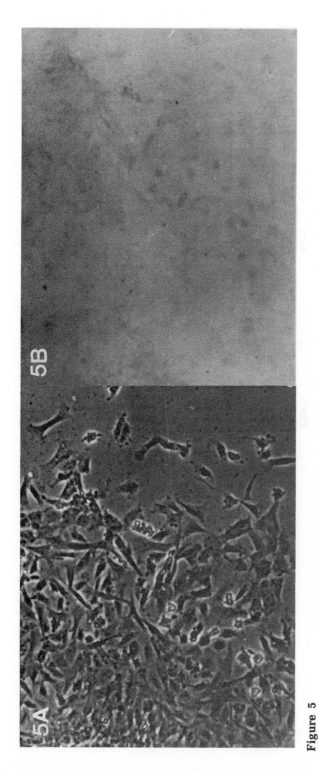

Figure 5
Staining of 2-day embryonic quail somitic mesenchymal cells by E/C8 monoclonal antibody (cultured for 24 hr prior to paraformaldehyde fixation). (A) Phase contrast; (B) bright-field illumination of cells in A.

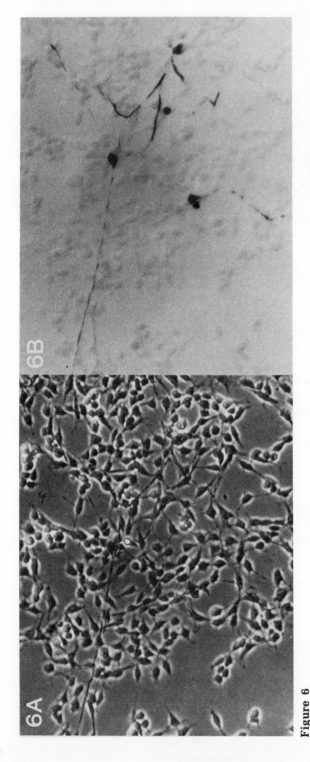

Figure 6
Staining of embryonic quail NC cells by E/C8 monoclonal antibody. Neural tubes from 2-day quail embryos were dissected and cultured for 2 days, during which time clusters of NC cells accumulated along the tube (see Loring et al. 1981). These clusters were removed with a tungsten needle, placed in individual wells of a 96-well plate, and allowed to attach and grow for 24 hr at 37°C. At that time, the cultures were paraformaldehyde-fixed. (A) Phase contrast; (B) bright-field illumination of cells in A.

Developmental Appearance of Antigen on Sensory and Sympathetic Neurons

"Squash" preparations of whole ganglia allow us to individualize all of the cells within the ganglion and to test their ability to bind various monoclonal antibodies. This technique not only allows us to count the total number of antigen-positive cells, but it also allows us to see the subcellular distribution of antigen on many cells within the ganglion.

In preliminary experiments, using E/C8-HRP on such preparations of chick sensory and sympathetic ganglia, we have observed that the initial pattern of neuronal staining is similar in both ganglionic types. After embryonic day 8, however, the antigen disappears on somata of sympathetic neurons and becomes more evenly distributed on somata of a subpopulation of sensory neurons. In both cell types, the antigen can be found on fibers at all stages examined.

In sensory ganglia of 7-day chick embryos, binding of E/C8-HRP is frequently confined to a region encompassing the initial segment of the neurite(s) and an adjacent patch on the cell soma. This pattern can be seen on most identifiable neurons at all developmental stages from bi- to unipolar cells (Tennyson 1965) (Fig. 7). At later developmental stages, the antigen can also be found on portions of the sensory neuronal somas distal to the neurite initial segment, so that by embryonic day 13 the antigen's presence is quite diffuse over the entire cell body.

In sympathetic ganglia of 7-day chick embryos (the earliest age used so far), the initial segment of the neurite and an adjacent patch on the neuronal soma stains (Fig. 8), as with sensory neurons. However, there are also occasional enclaves of cells that have intensely stained patches at one end of the cell but no discernible neurite (Fig. 8). If these are predifferentiated sympathetic neurons or neuroblasts, it is tempting to suggest that the stained region may be the site from which the neurite subsequently emerges. At later embryonic ages, the patches of staining on somata disappear and the proportion of antigen-positive cells without neurites is smaller, until by embryonic day 11 none could be found.

CONCLUSIONS

• In our initial attempts to address the question of lineages in NC sensory neuron development, we have presumed that some antigenic determinants may be confined to certain lineages or, possibly, to specific periods during a particular lineage development. If so, one

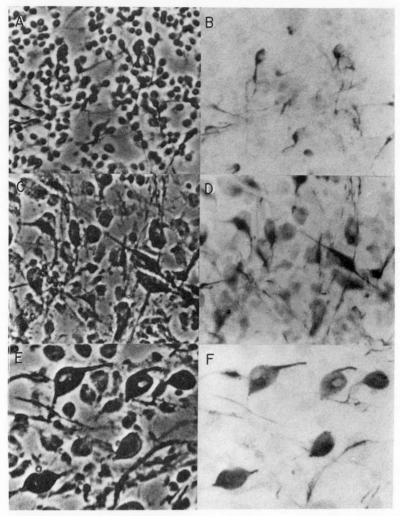

Figure 7
Staining by E/C8-HRP direct immunoperoxidase of squash preparations
using sensory ganglia from chick embryos of various ages. (A,B) 4-day
embryos; (C,D) 7-day embryos; (E,F) 11-day embryos. (A,C,E) Phase
contrast; (B,D,F) direct illumination of cells in A, C, and E, respectively.

might expect to find subpopulations of NC intermediate cells in
entirely different locales (e.g., embryonic sensory and sympathetic
ganglia) that express a common antigen and may in fact be developmentally equivalent. If this were so, they could be expected to give
rise to the same cell types if isolated and transplanted into identical

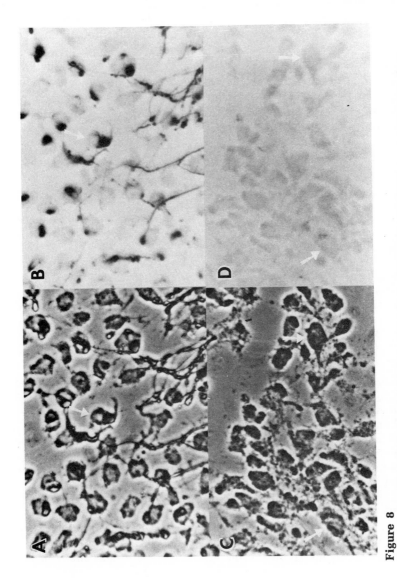

Figure 8
Staining by E/C8-HRP direct immunoperoxidase of squash preparations using sympathetic ganglia from chick embryos of various ages. (A,B) 7-day embryos; (C,D) 11-day embryos. (A,C) Phase contrast; (B,D) direct illumination of cells in A and C, respectively. (→) Presumed neurons.

environments. Several observations presented here are consistent with the notion that such lineages exist. These include the findings that (1) only subpopulations of sensory neurons stain with any of the antibodies developed, (2) subpopulations of NC cells also express these antigens (at least in culture), and (3) different neuronal derivatives of the NC may be initially similar in the expression of this phenotypic trait but seem to diverge after a particular developmental age.

The nature and biological functions of the antigens recognized by monoclonal antibodies raised in our lab are completely unknown. However, we hope that some of the antigens may be receptors for specific interactions involved in cellular differentiation. Antibodies to such determinants could then serve as molecular probes for analyzing and perturbing developmental regulatory events.

REFERENCES

Chalozonitis, A. and G.D. Fischbach. 1980. Elevated potassium induces morphological differentiation of dorsal root ganglionic neurons in dissociated cell culture. *Dev. Biol.* **78:**173.

Fields, K.L. 1979. Cell type-specific antigens of cells of the central and peripheral nervous system. *Curr. Top. Dev. Biol.* **13:**237.

Hamburger, V. and R. Levi-Montalcini. 1949. Proliferation, differentiation and degeneration in the spinal ganglia of the chick embryo under normal and experimental conditions. *J. Exp. Zoo.* **111:**457.

Hanker, J.S., P.E. Yates, C.B. Metz, and A. Rustioni. 1977. A new, specific, sensitive and noncarcinogenic reagent for the demonstration of horseradish peroxidase. *Histochem. J.* **9:**789.

Kauffman, S.A., R.M. Shymko, and K. Trabert. 1978. Control of sequential compartment formation in *Drosophila. Science* **199:**259.

Le Douarin, N.M. 1980. The ontogeny of the neural crest in avian embryo chimaeras. *Nature* **286:**663.

Le Douarin, N.M., M.A. Teillet, and C. Le Lievre. 1977. Influence of the tissue environment on the differentiation of neural crest cells. In *Cell and tissue interactions* (ed. J.W. Lash and M.M. Burger), p. 11. Raven Press, New York.

Le Douarin, N.M., M.A. Teillet, C. Ziller, and J. Smith. 1978. Adrenergic differentiation of cells of the cholinergic ciliary and Remak ganglia in avian embryo after *in vivo* transplantation. *Proc. Natl. Acad. Sci.* **75:**2030.

Loring, J., B. Glimelius, and J. Weston. 1979. Substrata of extracellular matrix (ECM) components affect the choice and expression of neural crest phenotypes. *J. Cell Biol.* **83:**41a.

Loring, J., B. Glimelius, C. Erickson, and J.A. Weston. 1981. Analysis of developmentally homogeneous neural crest cell populations *in vitro.* I. Formation, morphology, and differentiative behavior. *Dev. Biol.* **82:**86.

Nakane, P.K. and A. Kawaoi. 1974. Peroxidase labelled antibody. A new method of conjugation. *J. Histochem. Cytochem.* **22**:1084.

Nichols, D.H. and J.A. Weston. 1977. Melanogenesis in cultures of peripheral nervous tissue. I. The origin and prospective fate of cells giving rise to melanocytes. *Dev. Biol.* **60**:217.

Noden, D.M. 1978a. The control of avian cephalic neural crest cytodifferentiation. I. Skeletal and connective tissues. *Dev. Biol.* **67**:296.

————. 1978b. The control of avian cephalic neural crest cytodifferentiation. II. Neural tissues. *Dev. Biol.* **67**:313.

Nuttall, R.P. and N.K. Wessells. 1979. Veils, mounds, and vesicle aggregates in neurons elongating *in vitro*. *Exp. Cell Res.* **119**:163.

Patterson, P.H. 1978. Environmental determination of autonomic neurotransmitter functions. *Annu. Rev. Neurosci.* **1**:1.

Patterson, P.H. and L.L.Y. Chun. 1974. The influence of non-neuronal cells on catecholamine and acetylcholine synthesis and accumulation in cultures of dissociated sympathetic neurons. *Proc. Natl. Acad. Sci.* **71**:3607.

Shulman, M., C.D. Wilde, and G. Köhler. 1978. A better cell line for making hybridomas secreting specific antibodies. *Nature* **276**:269.

Tennyson, V.M. 1965. Electron microscopic study of the developing neuroblast of the dorsal root ganglion of the rabbit embryo. *J. Comp. Neurol.* **124**:267.

Tomozawa, Y. and N. Sueoka. 1978. *In vitro* segregation of different cell lines with neuronal and glial properties from a stem cell line of rat neurotumor RT4. *Proc. Natl. Acad. Sci.* **75**:6305.

Weston, J.A. 1970. The migration and differentiation of neural crest cells. *Adv. Morphog.* **8**:41.

————. 1981. Motile and social behavior of neural crest cells. In *The social abilities of cells* (ed. R. Bellairs et al.). Cambridge University Press, Cambridge, England. (In press.)

Monoclonal Antibodies Specific for Identifiable Leech Neurons

BIRGIT ZIPSER and RONALD McKAY
Cold Spring Harbor Laboratory
Cold Spring Harbor, New York 11724

• Nervous systems function through a series of precise contacts between neurons. There are two types of mechanisms that may account for the specificity of neuronal interaction. In one, the specificity of cell interaction is thought to be a consequence of neurons carrying a chemical label that determines the contacts (Sperry 1963). The second view suggests that initially neurons are not chemically predetermined but that specific networks are formed as a consequence of cell function (Weiss 1947). These two mechanisms are not mutually exclusive, and both explanations must postulate chemical differences between neurons that may remain in the adult functioning nervous system.

There is evidence from ultrastructural (Palay and Chan-Palay 1975) and physiological studies (Nicholls and Baylor 1968; Stuart 1970) that neurons are very diverse. Two other types of evidence are consistent with the idea that neurons as a class of cell are divided into a very heterogeneous number of subtypes. Immunohistochemical studies using antisera to neuropeptides reveal many different cell types among morphologically similar cells (Brecha et al. 1979), and studies of messenger RNA (mRNA) complexity from mammalian brain suggest that the nervous system as a whole requires the use of many more genes than do other organs (Hahn et al. 1978). However, mRNA complexity of cloned transformed cell lines with neuronal properties does not greatly exceed the complexity of other differentiated cell types. So the mRNA complexity of whole brain may be a consequence of many neural cell types.

These different lines of evidence support the view that neurons differ chemically from one another. Because these molecules are present in only a few cells and cannot be obtained in pure form, except in the case of neuropeptides, they are very difficult to study by traditional biochemical procedures. The description by Köhler and Milstein (1975) of an efficient method for cloning immunoglobulin (Ig)-secreting cells offers a promising solution to the problem of studying molecules that occur in only a few cells in a complex tissue.

Mice immunized with a histologically complex piece of nervous tissue will generate many antibodies to different antigens in this tissue. However, one Ig-secreting cell secretes only one antibody, and if we can grow this cell as a clonal population, we can study the properties of this antibody in isolation. The hybridoma technology permits many hundreds of Ig-secreting cell lines to be studied in this way. So, even though the molecules that characterize different neurons may be rare, we have a chance of finding them.

In this study we applied this strategy to the nervous system of the leech (Haemopis marmorata). Leeches are simple, segmented annelids. In each segment they have a ganglion containing a few hundred neuronal cell bodies (Fig. 1) that are connected (1) to the periphery by processes that grow out of the roots and (2) to other ganglia by axons that form the connective. A typical ganglion contains 400 neurons, and many of these cell bodies are bilaterally symmetrical. The structure of each ganglion is, in general, repeated in the next. Neurons in the leech are unipolar and synapse in a specialized region of each ganglion, the neuropil. At the head and tail of the animal, a number of ganglia have fused during evolution to form a larger structure. In addition, the head contains a structure, the supraesophageal ganglion, that may not be derived from the normal ectodermal lineage in development. The leech has two other advantages for this study, in addition to its anatomically simple structure: Many features of the leech's behavior are understood electrophysiologically (Muller 1979), and the embryological development of the nervous system is experimentally accessible (Weisblat et al. 1980).

Thus, in the leech we have an animal with a simple, reiterated nervous system in which many of the neurons have a defined function. The question we posed is, Can we use hybridoma technology to find antibodies that will bind only to specific neurons?

The nervous system was dissected out of a leech and used to immunize mice. After the hybridoma fusion, cells were plated into several hundred tissue culture wells. In one fusion we obtained 535 hybrid cell lines. We screened 475 of these for their ability to bind to whole-mount, detergent-permeabilized preparations of the leech nerve cord in an indirect immunofluorescence or immunoperoxidase screen. Of these, 300 cell lines secreted antibody that stained the nervous system. However, we identified 70 cell lines that gave interesting, nonuniform staining. Of these, 67 cell lines were grown and stored frozen.

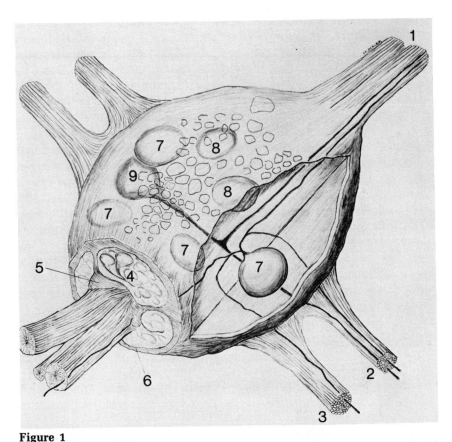

Figure 1

Diagram of a leech midbody ganglion. (1) Connective; (2) anterior root; (3) posterior root; (4) neuronal cell bodies in glial packages; (5) the beginning of the neuropil where synapses occur; (6) capsule; (7) two pairs of bilaterally symmetrical pressure cells; (8) the pair of large Retzius cells are shown in the background of several hundred neuronal cell bodies; (9) one of the two lateral penile evertor (PE) cells (the other has been dissected away). Each cell body has a characteristic location and number of axons. Note that the PE motor neuron projects into contralateral roots and that the sensory pressure cell has ipsilateral projections. Monoclonal antibodies were raised by immunizing mice with the entire leech nerve cord. Both the P3-X63-8Ag and SP2 cell lines were used as the myeloma parent. Hybrid cell lines were tested by direct immunohistochemical screening on the leech nerve cord. Interesting lines were cloned in soft agar. The leech nerve cords used in screening were fixed in 4% paraformaldehyde and 0.1 M phosphate buffer (pH 7.4) for 30 min at room temperature or in Bouin's fixative for 4 hr at room temperature. After washing in 0.05 M phosphate buffer (pH 7.4) and 0.9% sodium chloride, the connective-tissue capsules were cut; incubations with antibody and washes were in phosphate-buffered saline and 0.2% saponin.

Most of the hybridoma cell lines secreted antibodies that gave a uniform staining pattern. Some of the antibodies bind to antigens present in many neurons. An example of an antibody in this class is shown in Figure 2A. This antibody stained most of the cell bodies in a ganglion. The criterion used to select interesting antibodies was that they did not bind to all neurons in a ganglion. Figure 2, B and C, shows examples of antibodies of this type. Even though the cell bodies can be displaced when the ganglia are prepared for immunocytochemistry, many of the cell bodies stained in Figure 2 B and C clearly occur in symmetrical pairs.

Another type of specific staining occurs when a monoclonal antibody recognizes an antigenic determinant in the cell processes. Figure 3 shows two examples of this type of staining. In one case a bilaterally symmetrical fiber system is stained uniformly (Fig. 3B), and in another we see punctate staining (Fig. 3A), which is interpreted as indicating a discontinuous distribution of the antigenic determinant in another fiber system. The lack of stained cell bodies in the midbody ganglia shown in Figure 3 may be a consequence either of the lack of the determinant in the cell bodies or of the cell bodies of these fibers occurring at sites that have not been studied. In the case of the antigen recognized by the monoclonal antibody shown in Figure 3A, cell bodies containing the same or a cross-reacting antigenic determinant occur in the supraesophageal ganglion. The implication is that these cell bodies may send very long processes through the midbody ganglia.

In the leech many cells have known physiological functions. A group of neurons, the mechanosensory cells, are part of the reflex arcs

Figure 2
Antibodies binding to neuronal cell bodies. (A) Lan3-8; this monoclonal antibody stains most of the cell bodies in a midbody ganglion (indirect immunofluorescence, rhodamine-conjugated anti−mouse IgG as the second layer). (B) Lan2-1; this antibody stains many fewer cell bodies, including the pressure cells, which form part of the mechanosensory group (indirect immunoperoxidase staining, peroxidase-conjugated anti−mouse IgG as the second layer). (C) Lan3-2; this antibody stains only the four nociceptive cell bodies that occur in most midbody ganglia (indirect immunofluorescence, rhodamine-conjugated anti−mouse IgG as the second layer).

Figure 4
Three different monoclonal antibodies that stain the pressure cells: (A) Lan3-5; (B) Lan3-6; (C) Lan3-7. The pressure cells were identified by their morphology and, in two cases (A and B), by microinjection with lucifer yellow, followed by rhodamine-conjugated second antibody. (The three monoclonal antibodies were visualized by the indirect immunoperoxidase method.)

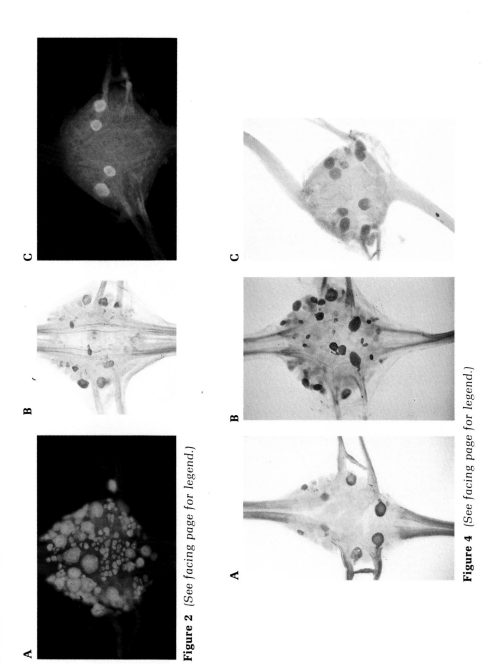

Figure 2 *(See facing page for legend.)*

Figure 4 *(See facing page for legend.)*

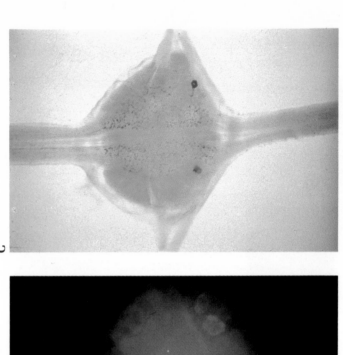

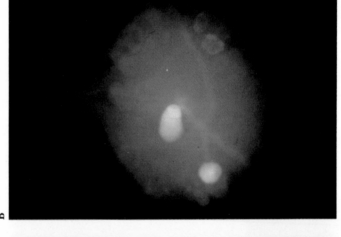

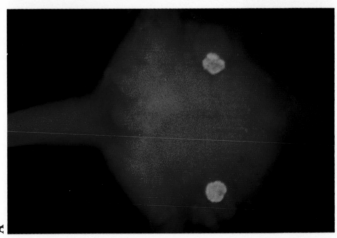

Figure 5 *(See facing page for legend.)*

that generate movement of the animal in response to stimulation of the body wall. This group contains cells of three types: those that respond to light touch, to pressure, and to nociceptive stimulation. One antibody specifically identifies the nociceptive cells (Fig. 1). Three monoclonal antibodies have been identified that bind to pressure cells (the staining patterns are shown in Fig. 4). Each of these antibodies, however, also stains other cell bodies, and each with a unique staining pattern. This result suggests that a single cell type, in this case the pressure cell, can carry a number of different specific antigenic markers.

These data show that there are a large number of antigenic determinants that occur on subgroups of neurons. This antigenic diversity is thought to reflect the different functions of neurons. We should be able to relate this molecular heterogeneity to the behavior of the animal.

Sexual behavior provides an example of a network that has been investigated by neurophysiological techniques in the leech (Zipser 1979a,b). About 20 different sex neurons have been identified by using backfill and electrophysiological techniques. Among them are two different pairs of neurons that are labeled by the antibody Lan3-1 (Fig. 5). The specific motor neuron character of the pair in ganglion 6 was determined in electrophysiological experiments; these are termed penile evertor (PE) cells. The specific function of the pair in ganglion 5 has yet to be established, although we already know that it is different. Thus, Lan3-1 binds to two different kinds of neurons subserving male reproductive function. These neurons not only belong to the larger sex network, but also to a particular sex subnetwork, as suggested by their close linkage through excitatory synaptic communication.

What makes the leech into a tractable preparation to study the molecular specificity of nerve cells is the possibility of identifying each neuron through a double-labeling experiment. The double-label-

Figure 5
(A) Lan3-1; by indirect immunofluorescence using rhodamine-conjugated antibody as the second layer, this monoclonal stains two large cell bodies in ganglia 5 and 6 (ganglion 6 is shown). (B) Before the immunofluorescence staining, the left lateral PE cell in the same ganglion as in Fig. 3A was identified physiologically and microinjected with lucifer yellow. One Retzius cell was also marked with lucifer yellow as a control (viewed here under fluorescein optics). (C) In all midbody ganglia, Lan3-1 stains two small cell bodies and varicosities in the neuropil. This staining is not evident in Fig. 5A since it occurs in a different focal plane from the PE cell (indirect immunoperoxidase staining).

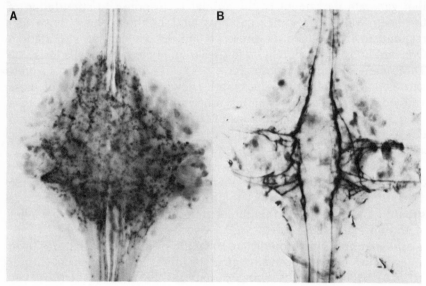

Figure 3
Monoclonal antibodies that bind to neuronal processes. (A) Lan3-9; in contrast to Lan2-3, this antibody stains a very large number of punctate varicosities. However, both antibodies are similar in that they fail to stain cell bodies in the midbody ganglia (indirect immunoperoxidase staining using the peroxidase-antiperoxidase procedure). (B) Lan2-3; this antibody detects a bilaterally symmetrical fiber system in each midbody ganglion.

ing technique, as indicated in Figure 5, combines intracellular dye injection with antibody staining. A cell body likely to be the antibody-labeled cell, as judged from its ganglionic location, diameter, and axonic projection, was impaled with a microelectrode under visual control. It was then characterized on the basis of its electrophysiological parameters and its synaptic relationships. The physiologically identified neuron was injected with lucifer yellow, and, as a control, another cell body, the Retzius cell, was also injected. The tissue was fixed and processed immunocytochemically, visualizing the monoclonal antibody through a rhodamine-coupled second antibody. In a successful double-labeling experiment, the identical cell body fluoresces yellow when viewed under fluorescein isothiocyanate (FITC) and red when viewed under rhodamine optics. Figure 5 shows that the same cell contains both the yellow fluorescent dye lucifer yellow and the antigen recognized by the monoclonal antibody Lan3-1. To establish the relationship between antigenicity and physiological networks, similar double-labeling experiments must be performed on all the cells identified by Lan3-1.

Several other types of neurons belong to the set of Lan3-1—labeled cells, as seen in Figure 5 and in the whole leech nerve cord

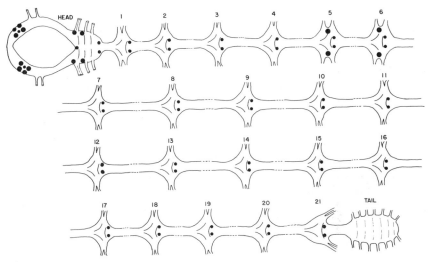

Figure 6
Map of Lan3-1 –positive cell bodies in the entire nerve cord of the leech. This diagram illustrates the symmetry and repetitive organization of this simple nervous system. The head map is still partial, and the tail ganglion also contains cell bodies, but their exact subganglionic location has not yet been determined.

diagram in Figure 6. Each midbody ganglion possesses a pair of smaller neurons, and additional cells are found in the head brains. We do not know whether or not these additional cells stained by Lan3-1 are part of the sex network. To determine whether the Lan3-1 antigen is solely shared by sex neurons requires screening for possible synaptic connections and other functional characteristics within the larger scope of the staining pattern.

CONCLUSION

• Monoclonal antibodies specific for identifiable leech neurons are produced by 5 –10% of the hybridoma clones tested. These antibodies have already proved themselves of value in broadening our understanding of leech neurobiology. For example, immunological identification of neurons is a convenient tool to help map variations in specific cell-body distributions along the entire leech nerve cord, a task that in the past was done solely with electrophysiological techniques. These findings show that groups of electrophysiologically distinct neurons are biochemically heterogeneous. This antigenic heterogeneity poses many questions. Among these are, Do functionally linked neurons share some antigenic markers, and are any of these antigens responsible for the specificity of neuronal connections?

REFERENCES

Brecha, N., H.J. Karten, and C. Laverack. 1979. Enkephalin-containing amacrine cells in the avian retina: Immunohistochemical localization. *Proc. Natl. Acad. Sci.* **76**:3010.

Hahn, W.C., J. Van Ness, and I.H. Maxwell. 1978. Complex population of mRNA sequences in large polyadenylated nuclear RNA molecules. *Proc. Natl. Acad. Sci.* **75**:5544.

Köhler, G. and C. Milstein. 1975. Continuous cultures of fused cells secreting antibody of predefined specificity. *Nature* **256**:495.

Muller, K.J. 1979. Synapses between neurones in the central nervous system of the leech. *Biol. Rev. Camb. Philos. Soc.* **54**:99.

Nicholls, J.G. and D.A. Baylor. 1968. Specific modalities and receptive fields of sensory neurons in CNS of the leech. *J. Neurophysiol.* **31**:740.

Palay, S.L. and V. Chan-Palay. 1975. A guide to the synaptic analysis of the neuropil. *Cold Spring Harbor Symp. Quant. Biol.* **40**:1.

Sperry, R.W. 1963. Chemoaffinity in the orderly growth of nerve fiber patterns and connections. *Proc. Natl. Acad. Sci.* **50**:703.

Stuart, A.D. 1970. Physiological and morphological properties of motoneurons in the central nervous system of the leech. *J. Physiol.* **209**:627.

Weisblat, D.A., G. Harper, G.S. Stent, and R.T. Sawyer. 1980. Embryonic cell lineages in the nervous system of the glossiphoniid leech *Helobdella triserialis*. *Dev. Biol.* **76**:58.

Weiss, P. 1947. Problem of specificity in growth and development. *Yale J. Biol. Med.* **19**:235.

Zipser, B. 1979a. Identifiable neurons controlling penile eversion in the leech. *J. Neurophysiol.* **42**:455.

————. 1979b. Voltage-modulated membrane resistance in coupled leech neurons. *J. Neurophysiol.* **42**:465.

Monoclonal Antibodies to Catecholamine-neurotransmitter-synthesizing Enzymes Can Be Used for Immunochemistry and Immunohistochemistry

M. ELIZABETH ROSS, EDWARD E. BAETGE, DONALD J. REIS, and TONG H. JOH

Cornell University Medical College
New York, New York 10021

• One of the important determinants of neurotransmitter availability is the activity of enzymes that subserve their biosynthesis. The activities and amounts of these enzymes are not fixed but are regulated by many factors, including substrate and cofactor availability, end-product concentration, nerve-impulse activity, and the hormonal and metabolic environment of the neuron. Specific antibodies against neurotransmitter-synthesizing enzymes are invaluable probes for the elucidation of mechanisms regulating these enzymes, particularly with reference to changes in their quantities, molecular forms, and turnover. Antibodies to these enzymes are also powerful tools for anatomical, morphological, and developmental characterization of neurons containing such specific markers.

By immunochemical titration, a change in enzyme activity triggered by neuronal injury, nerve stimulation, or drug administration can be shown to result from a change in the amount of enzyme present (induction or deinduction) (Joh et al. 1973; Reis et al. 1975; Ross et al. 1975) or a change in specific activity (activation) (Lewander et al. 1977). Using immunochemical trapping of enzyme into which isotopes have been incorporated during synthesis, relative rates of synthesis and degradation of the enzyme can be determined. More recently, we have begun to look at regulation of catecholamine-synthesizing enzymes from the vantage point of the nucleus. Specific antibodies can be used to isolate and quantitate a single gene product from in vitro translation of mRNA, purified from catecholamine-containing cells (Baetge et al. 1981). The combined capabilities of immunochemistry and molecular biology make possible examination

101

of intracellular regulation of neuronal function at its most fundamental levels.

We have used conventional rabbit antibodies for immunocytochemical localization and morphological studies of catecholamine-containing cells at both the light- and electron-microscopic levels (Pickel et al. 1976, 1978). They have been used in developmental studies for tracking the migration of catecholaminergic cells during embryogenesis as well as for describing the ontogeny of neurotransmitter synthesis in developing cells (Teitelman et al. 1979). Furthermore, transient populations of tyrosine (TH)-containing cells have been localized in kidney and pancreatic islets (Teitelman et al. 1981). In pancreas, using a double-labeling technique, these TH cells have been shown to differentiate into glucagon-secreting cells.

It is obvious that such advantageous uses of specific antibodies can be carried even further with monospecific antibodies. They could make it possible to identify isozymes possessing subtly different as well as common antigenic determinants. Moreover, it might be possible to obtain monoclonal antibodies to enzymes, such as choline acetyl transferase, for which it has been difficult to obtain highly specific conventional antisera or which have proved difficult to purify in quantities necessary for conventional immunization. The ability to provide a continuous and essentially unlimited supply of homogeneous, well-defined antibodies is an attractive feature of this approach. These considerations led us to produce hybridoma clones secreting monoclonal antibodies to dopamine-beta-hydroxylase (DBH) and TH (Ross et al. 1981).

GENERATION OF MONOCLONAL ANTIBODIES

• CB6 mice were sensitized either to partially purified rat striatal TH or bovine adrenal medullary DBH. Lymphocytes from these mice were fused with murine plasmacytoma NS1 cells. Spleen cells were used for feeder layers in culture. An enzyme-linked immunosorbant assay (ELISA) was employed to screen the hybridomas, of which 8 – 10% secreted the desired antibodies. Stable lines were established by limiting-dilution cloning. High antibody titers were obtained from ascites fluid of CB6 mice injected intraperitoneally with a single hybridoma clone.

CHARACTERIZATION OF ANTIBODIES

• Antibodies to DBH (CMD-6, -10, and -14) and TH (CMTH-29, -31, -78, and -95) were highly specific, as demonstrated both on ELISA, using enzyme antigen purified to homogeneity, and on immunoelectrophoresis, producing a single immunoprecipitin arc against homog-

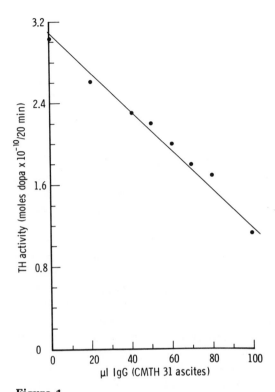

Figure 1
Immunotitration of TH from a crude extract of
rat caudate nucleus. Rat caudate nucleus was
homogenized (1 mg/30 μl) in 5 mM potassium
phosphate buffer (pH 7.0) with 0.2% Triton X-
100. After centrifugation at 10,000g for 15
min, increasing amounts of CMTH-31 IgG
from mouse ascites fluid were added to 20-μl
aliquots of the supernatant. Each mixture was
brought to a final volume of 120 μl in 0.9%
NaCl and incubated at room temperature for 1
hr. Then 20 μl of RAM was added to each
tube, and the samples were incubated for 30
min at room temperature. Precipitates were
sedimented at 27,000g for 15 min, and 50 μl
of each supernatant was assayed for TH
activity.

enates of bovine adrenal medulla (for CMDs [anti-DBH antibodies]) or
rat striatal tissue (for CMTHs [anti-TH antibodies]).

Alone, these antibodies failed to inhibit or fully precipitate DBH
or TH activity from solution. However, with the addition of rabbit
anti–mouse IgG (RAM), DBH-CMD or TH-CMTH complexes were

precipitated, thereby removing enzyme activity from solution. For example, by including RAM in the system, CMTH-31 linearly precipitated TH activity from a crude rat caudate nucleus extract, as shown in Figure 1.

In immunohistochemical studies, the TH monoclonal antibodies were found to tolerate fixation of preparations with 4% paraformaldehyde.

APPLICATIONS OF MONOCLONAL ANTIBODIES

• Using the peroxidase-antiperoxidase method for immunohistochemical localization of the enzyme, the CMTH antibodies afforded clear definition, with virtually no background staining, of perikarya, axons, and fine terminals in catecholamine-containing neurons throughout the rat brain (Fig. 2).

Recently, our laboratory has used anti-TH monoclonal antibodies (CMTH) to confirm our studies that determined that hormonally elicited increases in TH activity in pheochromocytoma (PC12) cells are due to an elevated rate of synthesis of the TH molecule, and not a decreased rate of degradation. At the molecular genetic level, TH was quantitated by immunoprecipitation from the products of in vitro translation of poly(A)$^+$ mRNA of control and dexamethasone-treated PC12 cells. PC12 cells were grown either in the presence or absence of dexamethasone. Poly(A)$^+$ mRNA was isolated from these cells by affinity chromatography on oligo(dT)-cellulose, translated in a reticulocyte-cell-free system in the presence of ^{3}H-labeled amino acids, and TH was immunoprecipitated. A fluorograph of the SDS-polyacrylamide gel electrophoresis of immunoprecipitated, ^{3}H-labeled protein revealed a band at the 60K molecular-weight position, corresponding to the subunit weight of authentic TH. Comparison of "control" and "dexamethasone-treated" systems showed that dexamethasone increases the translational activity of TH-mRNA approximately 2.5-fold in PC12 cells. Like the rabbit antiserum, monoclonal anti-TH antibodies (CMTH-78) precipitated the enzyme from products translated in vitro from purified poly(A)$^+$ mRNA and revealed the 2.5-

Figure 2
Immunohistochemical staining of TH in rat brain. IgG from culture supernatants was used in the peroxidase-antiperoxidase method as previously described (Teitelman et al. 1981). Each CMTH Ab (29, 31, 78, and 95) localized both noradrenergic and dopaminergic neurons in 30 μm sections. (A) Cell bodies of the locus ceruleus (surrounding tissue is counterstained with cresyl violet). Bar = 125 μm. (B) Perikarya of the locus subceruleus. Bar = 25 μm. (C) Cell bodies of substantia nigra. Bar = 100 μm. (D) Striato-nigral axons terminating in the caudate nucleus. Bar = 25 μm.

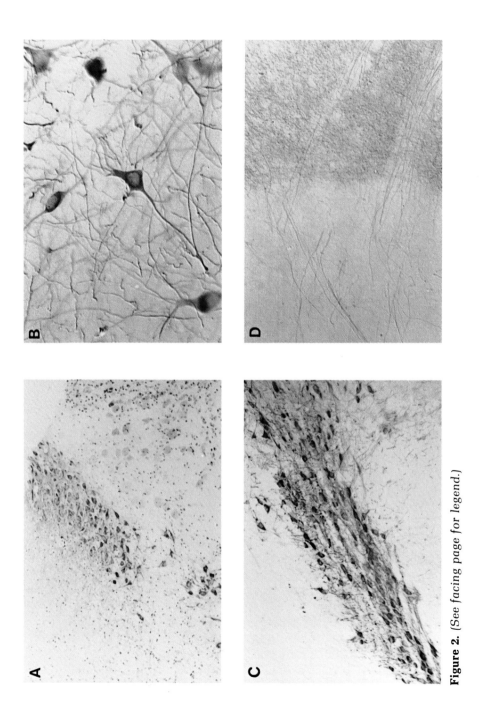

Figure 2. (See facing page for legend.)

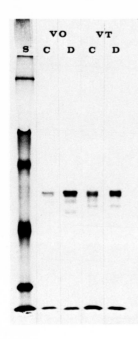

Figure 3

Fluorograph of immunoprecipitates, using CMTH-78 Ab, of TH synthesized in PC12 cells (VO) or translated from purified PC12 poly(A) mRNA (VT): effects of dexamethasone in culture media. PC12 cells were grown either in the presence (D) or absence (C) of dexamethasone for 3 days. One set of C and D cultures was then grown for 4 hr in a ^{3}H-labeled amino acid medium, collected and homogenized, and then ^{3}H-labeled TH was immunoprecipitated. Polysomes were prepared from the second set of control (C) and dexamethasone-treated (D) PC12 cells and poly(A) mRNA isolated by affinity chromatography on oligo(dT)-cellulose (Lewander et al. 1977). Poly(A) mRNA was translated in a reticulocyte system in the presence of ^{3}H-labeled amino acids, and TH was precipitated by CMTH-78 after the addition of RAM. This fluorograph of the SDS-polyacrylamide gel electrophoresis of the immunoprecipitated, ^{3}H-labeled protein shows, in each case, a major protein band of molecular weight 60,000 corresponding to authentic TH. (S) Standard proteins.

fold elevation in translation by dexamethasone (Fig. 3). Thus, TH has been unequivocally identified in our in vitro translation system. Whether this increased TH synthesis is controlled at the DNA (transcriptional) level or the mRNA level (an enhancement of translational efficiency) is a question that will be addressed when a copy DNA probe is developed.

CONCLUSION

• We have found that monoclonal antibodies to selected neurotransmitter-synthesizing enzymes are useful for: (1) quantitative immunoprecipitation of enzyme in tissues and cultured cells; (2) determination of rates of synthesis and degradation during enzyme induction; (3) isolation of enzymes from products translated in vitro from mRNA; and (4) immunocytochemical localization of enzymes in neural tissue. As more monospecific antibodies are produced against TH, DBH, and other neurotransmitter-synthesizing enzymes, we look forward to finding subtle antigenic differences among possible isozymes isolated from various tissues. By extending our repertoire of exquisitely specific antibodies, a broader range of neurotransmitter-synthesizing enzymes will be examined at the gene level. Furthermore, the ontogenesis of neuronal systems can be defined, and, using double-labeling techniques, possible interrelationships of these enzymes in the expression of genetic information of neurons will be closely studied in embryonic tissue.

ACKNOWLEDGMENT

• This work was supported by National Institutes of Health grants HL 18974 and MH 24285.

REFERENCES

Baetge, E.E., B.B. Kaplan, D.J. Reis, and T.H. Joh. 1981. Translation of tyrosine hydroxylase from poly(A) mRNA in pheochromocytoma cells (PC12) is enhanced by dexamethasone. *Proc. Natl. Acad. Sci.* **78**:1269.

Joh, T.H., C. Geghman, and D.J. Reis. 1973. Immunochemical demonstration of increased accumulation of tyrosine hydroxylase protein in sympathetic ganglia and adrenal medulla elicited by reserpine. *Proc. Natl. Acad. Sci.* **70**:2767.

Lewander, T., T.H. Joh, and D.J. Reis. 1977. Tyrosine hydroxylase: Delayed activation in central noradrenergic neurons and induction in adrenal medulla elicited by stimulation of central cholinergic receptors. *J. Pharmacol. Exp. Ther.* **200**:523.

Pickel, V.M., T.H. Joh, and D.J. Reis. 1976. Monoamine-synthesizing enzymes in central dopaminergic, noradrenergic, and serotonergic neurons: Immunocytochemical localization by light and electron microscopy. *J. Histochem. Cytochem.* **24**:792.

Pickel, V.M., T.H. Joh, D.J. Reis, S.E. Leeman, and R.J. Miller. 1978. Electron microscopic localization of substance P and enkephalin in axon terminals related to dendrites of catecholaminergic neurons. *Brain Res.* **158**:229.

Reis, D.J., T.H. Joh, and R.A. Ross. 1975. Effects of reserpine on activities and amounts of tyrosine hydroxylase and dopamine-beta-hydroxylase in catecholaminergic neuronal systems in rat brain. *J. Pharmacol. Exp. Ther.* **193**:775.

Ross, R.A., T.H. Joh, and D.J. Reis. 1975. Reversible changes in the accumulation and activities of tyrosine hydroxylase and dopamine-beta-hydroxylase in neurons of nucleus locus ceruleus during the retrograde reaction. *Brain Res.* **92**:57.

Ross, M.E., D.J. Reis, and T.H. Joh. 1981. Monoclonal antibodies to tyrosine hydroxylase: Production and characterization. *Brain Res.* **208**:493.

Teitelman, G., T.H. Joh, and D.J. Reis. 1981. Transformation of catecholaminergic precursors into glucagon "A" cells in the mouse embryonic pancreas. *Proc. Natl. Acad. Sci.* (in press).

Teitelman, G., H. Baker, T.H. Joh, and D.J. Reis. 1979. Appearance of catecholamine synthesizing enzymes during development of rat sympathetic nervous system: Possible role of tissue environment. *Proc. Natl. Acad. Sci.* **76**:509.

Monoclonal Antibodies to Neurotransmitter Substances

A. CLAUDIO CUELLO

Department of Pharmacology and Human Anatomy
University of Oxford
Oxford, England OX1 3QT

CESAR MILSTEIN

Medical Research Council
Laboratory of Molecular Biology
Cambridge, England CB2 2QH

• The understanding of brain function largely depends on the knowledge of the fine anatomy of transmitter-specific synapses. As an example, areas of processing of primary sensory information are now known to display a number of peptide-containing and amine-containing fibers. Peptide-peptide and amine-peptide interactions have been postulated there.

In spite of the rapidly growing information on the occurrence of neuroactive substances in the peripheral afferents and in local circuit and projecting neurons in these areas, little is known of their defined synaptic interactions. The discovery that amines and peptides can coexist in neurons that project to these areas further complicates the situation.

We are currently developing monoclonal antibodies to neurotransmitter and related substances, aiming toward the elucidation of some of these transmitter-specific synaptic interactions. New techniques, including internal radiolabeling of monoclonal antibodies, are being developed to achieve the simultaneous demonstration of multiple transmitter-related antigens at cellular and subcellular levels, particularly in relation to the possible coexistence of neurotransmitter substances in single neurons of the central nervous system (CNS).

Neurotransmitter substances are usually poor antigens, sometimes even when conjugated to carrier proteins. Conventional sera, when successfully obtained, will vary considerably from animal to animal, and even from bleed, to bleed with regard to characteristics and affinity as well as relative abundance of individual antibody molecules. The hybridoma technique can immortalize specific antibodies and enables their wide distribution as standard reagents. This is even more advantageous in studies of neurotransmitter localization when large amounts of antibodies are required.

Internal labeling of monoclonal antibodies with radioactive amino acids to a high specific acivity offers a number of advantages in immunocytochemistry. In contrast to external labeling, internal labeling is free from partial or severe inactivation of antibody. Radiographic detection and localization of antigens can be achieved at both light and electron microscopic levels. The fact that complexes of secondary antibodies and enzymic reaction products are obviated render better penetration and better preserved ultrastructure in the preparation. In addition, autoradiographic grains do not obscure the subjacent subcellular features.

We here describe our monoclonal antibodies to substance P and serotonin and demonstrate the coexistence of these substances in a single neuron by combined use of immunoenzyme technique and autoradiography of an internally labeled monoclonal antibody.

GENERATION AND RADIOLABELING OF MONOCLONAL ANTIBODIES

• Monoclonal antibody to substance P (NC1/34-HL) was developed from a fusion of NS1 cells with spleen cells of Wistar rats immunized with substance P conjugated to bovine serum albumin (Cuello et al. 1979). Clones were screened for the presence of anti–substance P antibodies by radioimmunoassay involving radioiodinated [Tyr^8]substance P. NC1/34-HL antibody recognizes the C-terminal portion of substance P with very high specificity. With this antibody it was possible to develop a radioimmunoassay that can detect down to 10 fmoles of substance P per tube.

Monoclonal antibody to serotonin (YC5/45-HLK) was obtained from a fusion of a rat myeloma line (Y3-Ag-1.2.3) and spleen cells of a rat immunized with serotonin-seroalbumin conjugate (A. Consolazione et al., in prep.). This antibody recognizes 5HT-containing sites in the formaldehyde-fixed preparations of the CNS.

Both monoclonal antibodies have been applied as primary antibodies in immunocytochemistry in conjunction with the indirect immunofluorescence technique for light microscopy studies and with the peroxidase-antiperoxidase technique (Sternberger et al. 1970) for light and electron microscopy studies.

NC1/34-HL antibody has been used as the redissolved ammonium sulfate precipitate from the culture fluid. Similar material has been used from supernatant of YC5/45 and also from bleedings from various strains of rats into which the clone was injected and grown as a tumor.

Internal radiolabeling of NC1/34-HL antibody (anti–substance P) was accomplished by incubating the cloned hybrid cells in medium containing 1 to 5 mCi of [³H]lysine. The culture medium was dialyzed against large volumes of phosphate-buffered saline. The radioactive reagent obtained had a specific radioactivity ranging from 300 to 2000 Ci/mmole of antibody. These antibodies have been used as radioimmunological probes to detect intracellular antigenic sites in light microscopy and high-resolution autoradiography (Cuello et al. 1980).

IMMUNOCYTOCHEMISTRY OF SUBSTANCE P AND 5HT USING MONOCLONAL ANTIBODIES

• The application of NC1/34-HL in light microscopy has confirmed the presence of substance P in specific areas of the CNS (Fig. 1). Lesion studies and administration of drugs have revealed organiza-

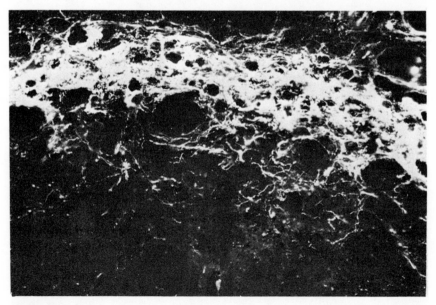

Figure 1
Substance P immunoreactive sites in the lower medulla oblongata of the rat as revealed by NC1/34-HL (mouse × rat) monoclonal antibody developed with the indirect immunofluorescence technique. The dense fluorescent bands represent fibers and nerve terminals over the substantia gelatinosa of the spinal nucleus of the trigeminal nerve. Note individual fibers with varicosities over the spinal (top) and nucleus propius of the trigeminal nerve.

tion and functional aspects of this peptide in the CNS and periphery (Cuello et al. 1980; Del Fiacco and Cuello 1980; Costa et al. 1980). The use of this monoclonal antibody for electron microscopy immunocytochemical studies in the trigeminal system (Fig. 2) and in the substantia nigra provided a detailed account of the synaptology of the substance-P-containing neurons in areas involved in nociception and in striatal circuits. This antibody also allowed us to confirm the presence of this peptide in defined primary sensory neurons (Cuello et al. 1980), striatal neurons (Cuello 1981), enteric neurons (Del Fiacco and Cuello 1980), and local circuit neurons of the retina (Karten and Brecha 1979).

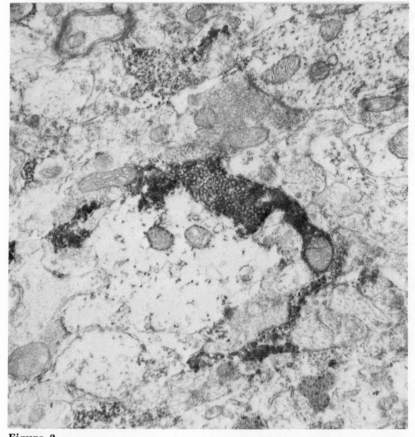

Figure 2
Electron micrograph showing a substance P immunoreactive nerve terminal (dark profile) surrounding a large dendrite in the substantia gelatinosa of the spinal nucleus of the trigeminal nerve. The anti−substance P monoclonal antibody (NC1/34-HL) has been developed with a rat peroxidase-antiperoxidase complex.

The YC5/45-HLK allowed the identification of the 5HT-containing cell bodies in the raphe nuclei system (Fig. 3). This immunostaining disappeared after the administration of PCPA, an inhibitor of

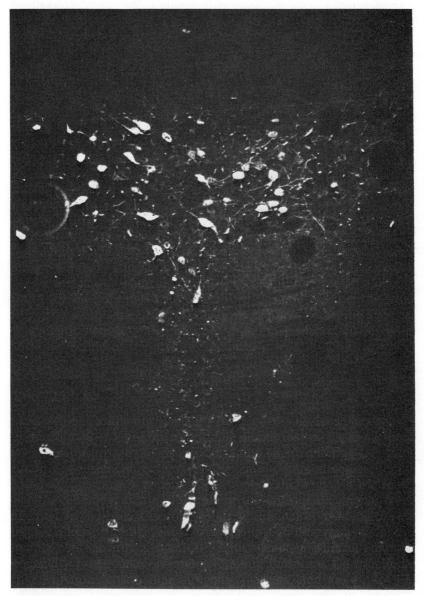

Figure 3
Serotonin immunoreactive neurons in the dorsal raphe nucleus of the rat as revealed by a rat × rat monoclonal antibody (YC5/45-HLK) and developed with an indirect immunofluorescence technique.

tryptophan hydroxylase, and is not affected by α-methyl-p-tyrosine, an inhibitor of tyrosine hydroxylase.

The use of internally radiolabeled monoclonal antibody (^{3}H-labeled NC1/34-HL) for detecting substance P provided an alternative to indirect techniques to detect this peptide (Fig. 4). This antibody has also been successfully applied for high-resolution autoradiography at the electron microscopic level (Fig. 5). The most outstanding aspect of this new application is the remarkable ultrastructural preservation of the tissue in contrast to the usual immunoenzyme techniques.

By combining autoradiography (for ^{3}H-labeled NC1/34-HL, anti—substances P) and the peroxidase-antiperoxidase technique (for YC5/45-HLK, anti-5HT) at the light microscopy level, it has been possible to stain simultaneously for substance P and serotonin and to show the coexistence of these two neuroactive substances in single neurons in the nucleus raphe magnus of the rat. Owing to a high specific radioactivity of the antibody, 3-day exposure was adequate for autoradiography in this experiment. We are currently exploring the combined use at both the light and electron microscopy levels of other antibodies developed with immunoenzyme methodology (Fig. 6).

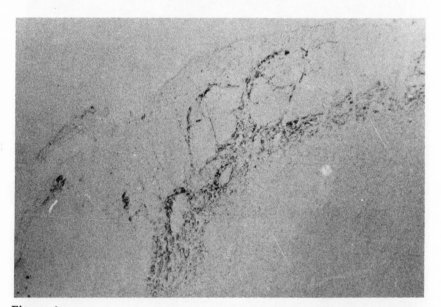

Figure 4
Autoradiography of a section of the rat medulla oblongata incubated with internally labeled anti—substance P monoclonal antibody (^{3}H-labeled NC1/34-HL). The dark band is composed of silver grains showing the presence of radioactive antibodies bound to nerve terminals in the substantia gelatinosa of the trigeminal nerve and over incoming primary sensory fibers (top).

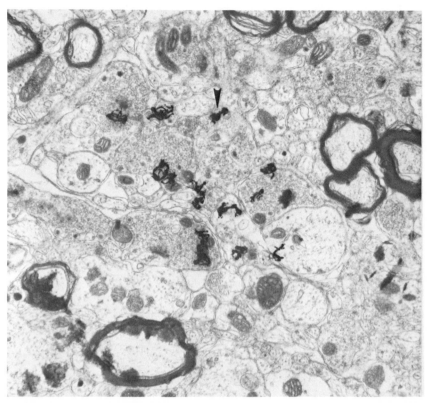

Figure 5
High-resolution autoradiograph illustrating the use of internally labeled monoclonal antibody (³H-labeled NC1/34-HL) for the localization of substance P immunoreactive sites. Silver grains (e.g., see arrowhead) denote the presence of bound antibodies over nerve terminals.

CONCLUSION

• Monoclonal antibodies to substance-P- and 5HT-containing sites were obtained and used in immunocytochemical localization of these antigenic sites in the rat nervous system. Anti−substance P monoclonal antibody was internally radiolabeled with tritium to a high specific activity. This antibody allowed high-resolution autoradiographic immunocytochemistry and illustrated the advantages of internally labeled antibodies. By combining autoradiography and the peroxidase-antiperoxidase technique, the coexistence of substance P and serotonin in single neurons was demonstrated. It is hoped that the unique possibilities of the application of monoclonal antibodies will

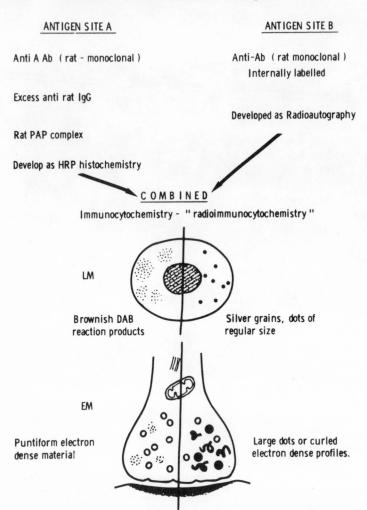

ANTIGEN SITE A

Anti A Ab (rat - monoclonal)

Excess anti rat IgG

Rat PAP complex

Develop as HRP histochemistry

ANTIGEN SITE B

Anti-Ab (rat monoclonal)
Internally labelled

Developed as Radioautography

COMBINED

Immunocytochemistry - " radioimmunocytochemistry "

LM

Brownish DAB
reaction products

Silver grains, dots of
regular size

EM

Puntiform electron
dense material

Large dots or curled
electron dense profiles.

Figure 6
Scheme illustrating the principle of the technique developed
for the simultaneous detection of two antigenic sites, A and B,
using monoclonal antibodies, revealed with the immunoenzyme procedure (for antigen A) and with autoradiography for
the internally labeled antibody (for antigen B). (*LM*) Light
microscopy; (*EM*) electron microscopy; (*PAP*) peroxidase antiperoxidase; (*HRP*) horseradish peroxidase; (*DAB*) 3,3'-
diaminobenzidine.

make important contributions to the understanding of the synaptic
relations between transmitter-specific neurons as well as of the coexistence of neuroactive substances in single neurons.

REFERENCES

Chan-Palay, V., G. Jonsson, and S.L. Palay. 1978. Serotoxin and substance P coexist in neurons of the rat's central nervous system. *Proc. Natl. Acad. Sci.* **75**:1582.

Cuello, A.C. 1981. Peptidergic neurones in striatal circuits. In *Regulatory functions of CNS* (ed. J. Szenthagothai and J. Hamori). Pergamon Press, Oxford. (In press.)

Cuello, A.C. 1981. Peptidergic neurones in striatal circuits. In *Regulatory functions of CNS* (ed. J. Szenthagothai and J. Hamori), Pergamon Press, Oxford. (In press.)

Cuello, A.C., G. Galfre, and C. Milstein. 1979. Detection of substance P in the central nervous system by a monoclonal antibody. *Proc. Natl. Acad. Sci.* **76**:3532.

Cuello, A.C., C. Milstein, and J.V. Priestley. 1980. Use of monoclonal antibodies in immunocytochemistry with special reference to the central nervous system. *Brain Res. Bull.* **5**:575.

Cuello, A.C., R. Gamse, P. Holzer, and F. Lembeck. 1981. Substance-P immunoreactive neurons following neonatal administration of capsaicin. *Naunyn-Schmieden bergs Arch. Pharmacol.* **315**:185.

Del Fiacco, M. and A.C. Cuello. 1980. Substance P and enkephalin-containing neurones in the rat trigeminal system. *Neuroscience* **5**:803.

Hökfelt, T., A. Ljungdahl, H. Steinbusch, A. Verhofstad, G. Nilsson, E. Brodin, B. Pernow, and M. Goldstein. 1978. Immunohistochemical evidence of substance P–like immunoreactivity in some 5-hydroxtryptamine-containing neurones in the rat central nervous system. *Neuroscience* **3**:517.

Karten, H.J. and N. Brecha. 1979. Localization of substance P immunoreactivity in amacrine cells of the retina. *Nature* **283**:87.

Sternberger, L.A., P.H. Hardy, Jr., J.J. Cuculis, and H.G. Meyer. 1970. The unlabeled antibody enzyme method of immunochemistry. Preparation and properties of soluble antigen-antibody complex (horseradish peroxidase-antihorseradish peroxidase) and its use in identification of spirochetes. *J. Histochem. Cytochem.* **18**:315.

Identification of a Polypeptide Specific to the Rat Nervous System

RICHARD AKESON, JANE S. RODMAN, KAREN GRAHAM, and ALICE ROBERTS

Institute for Developmental Research
Children's Hospital Research Foundation
Cincinnati, Ohio 45229

• In the development and functioning of the nervous system, cells are governed by both their genetic phenotype and their environment, including other cells. Response to and interaction with the environment may be mediated by specific components on the surfaces of the cells. Our objective is to identify such molecules and to analyze their roles in the mechanisms that govern the development of the nervous system.

Immunological technology, particularly with monoclonal antibodies, has the promise of providing very specific probes to detect, quantitate, and localize the individual cell-surface components. Antibodies offer the further utility of potentially compromising the function(s) of such molecules both in vitro (Buskirk et al. 1980) and in vivo (Costa et al. 1979; Williams et al. 1980), thus giving clues to the functions of such molecules as well as to their chemical identities.

Thus, we are attempting to produce monoclonal antibodies to neural antigens found early in development or on restricted classes of neurons. Tumor cell lines of neural origin are convenient immunogens for such a purpose (Stallcup and Cohn 1976) since they offer a uniform population of cells expressing surface antigens that may be relatively rare components in nervous tissue. We describe here a monoclonal antibody that we obtained, G5-IgG, and report our studies on the chemical nature, distribution, and biological function of G5 antigen.

GENERATION OF THE MONOCLONAL ANTIBODY G5-IgG

• BALB/c mice were immunized with three intraperitoneal injections of 5 × 10⁶ to 6 × 10⁶ PC12 cells. X63 myeloma cells were used for fusion. The hybrid clones were screened for production of antibodies that bind to adult rat brain particulate protein in a microfuge precipitation assay involving radioiodinated protein A. The hybrid clone G5 was obtained from one of several positive wells and recloned. Interestingly, the monoclonal antibody G5-IgG did not bind to PC12 cells or any other cultured rat cell lines tested.

TISSUE DISTRIBUTION OF G5 ANTIGEN

• G5-IgG reacts with particulate protein preparations from adult rat brain, spinal cord, and retina but not adrenal in a ^{125}I-labeled protein-A binding assay. Some binding is also seen with the immune system tissues bone marrow, spleen, and spleen capsule but not lymph node, thymus, or thymus capsule (Akeson and Graham 1981). A small amount of binding is observed with lung (presumably due to lymphoid contamination) but none is seen with heart, kidney, liver, ovary, skeletal muscle, or epididymal sperm. Brain binds 10 to 100 times more G5-IgG per milligram protein than any other tissue tested. Thus, analysis of whole organs indicates that G5-IgG detects a nervous system antigen that is also found in substantially reduced levels on some lymphoid cells.

Springer et al. (1979) detected a mouse macrophage surface antigen Mac-1 with a monoclonal antibody that precipitates components of 190,000 and 105,000 daltons. The G5 antigen appears to be distinct from Mac-1 since the latter was not detected in mouse brain and because G5-IgG exhibited more activity toward nonadherant fractions compared with adherant fractions from the peritoneal exudate cells of glycogen-primed rats. The fact that the spleen capsule showed a higher activity than the spleen suggests that G5 antigen may be associated with precursor cells in the immune system.

MOLECULAR NATURE OF G5 ANTIGEN

• Chemical characterization was done with G5 antigen solubilized in a buffer containing 0.5% NP-40. The antigen was assayed by its ability to inhibit the binding of G5-IgG to a glutaraldehyde-fixed rat brain particulate protein preparation.

The antibody binding was not inhibited by a 3 M KCl extract or a chloroform-methanol extract. When the immunoprecipitate from a radioiodinated and detergent-solubilized particulate preparation was analyzed by Laemmli-type SDS electrophoresis, a single band in the region of molecular weight 95–105K was detected (Fig. 1). This band

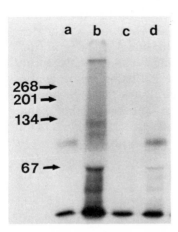

Figure 1

Autoradiographs of immunoprecipitates of ^{125}I-labeled NP-40-solubilized adult rat brain particulate protein electrophoresed on SDS-polyacrylamide gels. Immunoglobulins used were G5-IgG (a), X63-"IgG" (b), G5-IgG adsorbed with rat brain (c), and G5-IgG adsorbed with rat liver (d).

was absent when control peritoneal fluid was used, or when the antibody was preabsorbed with a rat brain particulate fraction, but was present when preabsorbed with a liver particulate fraction. When the immunoprecipitate was analyzed without reduction, a single band was detected in the same position, indicating the lack of an intermolecular disulfide bond in situ. Since G5 antigen was not detectable in an electrophoretic analysis of total radioiodinated particulate fraction, it is not a major membrane component.

When material solubilized by NP-40 was incubated with concanavalin A–sepharose beads, activity inhibiting antibody binding was

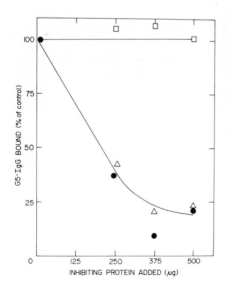

Figure 2

The effect of concanavalin A–agarose beads on the ability of NP-40-solubilized rat brain particulate protein to inhibit G5-IgG binding. Solubilized brain particulate protein was preincubated with concanavalin A beads (□) or concanavalin A beads plus 0.1 M α-methyl mannopyranoside (Δ) or mock incubated (▲). The supernatant was tested for its ability to inhibit binding of G5-IgG to glutaraldehyde-fixed rat brain.

removed (Fig. 2). This removal was not observed in the presence of α-methyl pyranoside, indicating that G5 antigen is either glycosylated or is closely associated with some glycosylated moiety. When an unlabeled immunoprecipitate was collected using Staph A, analyzed on a Laemmli-type gel, and developed with radioiodinated concanavalin A, a band at 90–95K (see arrowhead on Fig. 3) was present, indicating the G5 molecule is itself glycosylated. The only other band present appears at 55K and can be ascribed to the IgG heavy chain, which is known to be glycosylated.

Thus, the G5 antigen appears to be a glycoprotein with characteristics of a monomolecular integral membrane component (Rodman and Akeson 1981).

BIOLOGY OF G5 ANTIGEN

• A first step in understanding the function(s) of the G5 antigen is the identification of cell type(s) that carry this molecule. Since no cultured cell line reacted with G5-IgG, primary cultures were tested for binding of G5-IgG, using immunofluorescence. Primary cultures from rat cerebrum and cerebellum from newborn and 4-day-old animals were largely negative. Occasional cells were positive, but as yet we have not been able consistently to obtain positive cultures for definite identification of the G5-positive cells.

Immunohistochemical localization of G5 antigen in cryostat sections of the rat cerebellum was attempted using radioiodinated pro-

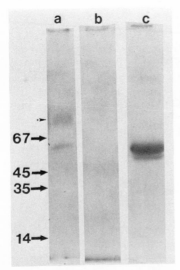

Figure 3
Visualization of rat brain immunoprecipitates using ^{125}I-labeled concanavalin A. Immunoprecipitates between unlabeled NP-40-solubilized rat brain particulate protein and G5-IgG (a) or X63-"IgG" (b) were electrophoresed in SDS gels and then soaked in ^{125}I-labeled-concanavalin A. G5-IgG alone was run as a control (c).

tein A and autoradiography. In the adult, G5 antigen was found almost exclusively in the molecular layer. The antigen was also detected in the cerebrum, but without the precise layering found in the cerebellum.

The molecular layer develops postnatally. Analysis of G5 expression in whole brain from rats of various ages indicated that it also develops postnatally (Fig. 4). Induction of this expression could be due to the postnatal birth of new cell types, interaction among cell types, or other factors.

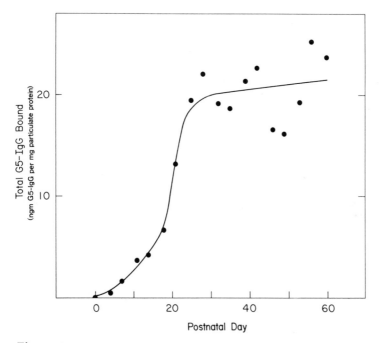

Figure 4

Content of G5 antigen in whole rat brain of various ages. Particulate protein preparations were assayed in the antibody-excess assay (Rodman and Akeson 1981) to determine total G5 content. Briefly increasing amounts of peritoneal fluid from BALB/c mice carrying G5 tumor or IgG preparations therefrom were reacted with 100 μg of particulate protein to determine a saturation curve and thus antigen-antibody equivalence. Bound antibody was detected with excess ^{125}I-labeled protein A from *Staphylococcus aureus*. Subsequent assays were performed with three times the equivalence amount of antibody for cerebral cortex, the tissue with highest activity. Control experiments used equivalent volumes of peritoneal fluid from mice carrying the parent X63 myeloma.

CONCLUSIONS AND PROSPECTS

• A monoclonal antibody (G5-IgG) to a rat neural antigen (G5) was obtained and used to study the distribution and molecular nature of this antigen. Brain has the highest activity of G5, with lesser amounts in some neural and immune tissues. G5 is an integral membrane glycoprotein with a molecular weight of 95–105K. Further attempts are being made to establish the cell-type specificity and to study the regulation of expression of the antigen. A possible role in cell-cell interaction in the developing postnatal brain is suggested by the detection in synaptosomes of a peptide with similar characteristics (Rodman and Akeson 1981). The extensive information accumulated on cerebellar development makes it a favorable system within which to determine the role of individual components in the cellular interactions necesssary for the development of the nervous system.

REFERENCES

Akeson, R. and K.L. Graham. 1981. A new antigen common to the rat nervous and immune systems. I. Detection with a hybridoma. *J. Neurosci. Res.* **6:** (in press).

Buskirk, D.R., J.P. Thiery, U. Rutishauser, and G.M. Edelman. 1980. Antibodies to a neural cell adhesion molecule disrupt histogenesis in cultured chick retina. *Nature* **285:**488.

Costa, M., L.B. Geffen, R.A. Rush, D. Bridges, W.W. Blessing, and J.W. Heath. 1979. Immune lesions of central noradrenergic neurons produced by antibodies to dopamine-β-hydroxylase. *Brain Res.* **173:**65.

Greene, L.A. and A.S. Tischler. 1976. Establishment of a noradrenergic clonal line of rat adrenal pheochromocytoma cells which respond to nerve growth factor. *Proc. Natl. Acad. Sci.* **73:**2424.

Rodman, J.S. and R. Akeson. 1981. A new antigen common to the rat nervous and immune systems. II. Molecular characterization. *J. Neurosci. Res.* **6:** (in press).

Springer, T., G. Galfre, D.S. Secher, and C. Milstein. 1979. Mac-1: A macrophage differentiation antigen identified by monoclonal antibody. *Eur. J. Immunol.* **9:**301.

Stallcup, W.B. and M. Cohn. 1976. Correlation of surface antigens and cell type in cloned cell lines from the rat cultured nervous system. *Exp. Cell Res.* **98:**285.

Williams, C.A., J. Barna, and N. Schupf. 1980. Antibody to Thy-1 antigen injected into rat hypothalamus selectively inhibits carbamyl choline induced drinking. *Nature* **283:**82.

A Monoclonal Antibody Recognizes a Determinant Present on Common As Well As Class-specific Intermediate Filament Subunits

REBECCA M. PRUSS,* RHONA MIRSKY, and MARTIN C. RAFF
Neuroimmunology Group
Department of Zoology
University College London
London, England WC1E 6BT

ROBIN THORPE and BRIAN H. ANDERTON
St. George's Hospital Medical School
London, England SW17 ORE

• Intermediate filaments are cytoskeletal components of most animal cells (Lazarides 1980). Although the filaments present in different cell types are morphologically similar, with a typical diameter of about 10 nm, they have been divided into five classes based on the cell type they are associated with, subunit composition, and immunochemical properties (Table 1).

Two intermediate filament classes are specific to the nervous system: (1) neurofilaments, which are found in central and peripheral neurons, and which in vertebrates are composed of three subunits with molecular weights of about 200K, 150K, and 70K; and (2) glial filaments, which are found in astroglia and contain a 50K protein known as glial fibrillary acidic protein (GFAP).

Three other intermediate filament classes are: (1) desmin filaments, present in muscles and composed of a 52K protein; (2) keratin filaments, or tonofilaments, specific to epithelial cells, with a family of polypeptides of molecular weight in the 47–68K range; and (3)

*Present address: Laboratory of Clinical Science, National Institute of Mental Health, National Institutes of Health, Bethesda, Maryland 20205

Table 1
Classes of Intermediate Filaments

Filament type	Cell type associated with	Subunits	Molecular weight
Neurofilament	neuron		200K, 150K, 70K (vertebrate)
Glial filament	astrocyte	GFAP	50K
Desmin-type filament	muscle cell	desmin	52K
Keratin-type filament (tonofilament)	epithelial cell	keratin	a family of polypeptides ~47–68K
Vimentin-type filament	many cell types	vimentin	58K + others

vimentin filaments with a subunit molecular weight around 52–58K, found in fibroblasts as well as in other cell types either alone or in combination with one of the other four classes of intermediate filaments.

We have previously obtained a rabbit antiserum to GFAP and found it to specifically label cultured astrocytes (Pruss 1979; Raff et al. 1979). To extend this approach, we wished to identify more antisera that specifically labeled different cell types in the nervous system. At the same time it was important to raise antisera in different species, so as to allow double labeling by the indirect immunofluorescence technique. Since we had a good rabbit antiserum against GFAP, we tried to raise such sera in mice. This was difficult even when a number of different strains of mice were tried, and when they did produce antibodies, they were very unstable. We therefore utilized the hybridoma technique to generate a continuous source of mouse anti-GFAP for use in immunocytochemical studies.

Figure 1
Double labeling of cultured cells from rat corpus callosum using the monoclonal antibody and rabbit anti-GFAP. Cells were fixed with acid ethanol prior to incubation with hybridoma supernatant overnight at 4°C. Cells were subsequently labeled using goat anti–mouse immunoglobulin (G anti-MIg) coupled with rhodamine (Rd), followed by rabbit anti-GFAP and then goat anti–rabbit immunoglobulin (G anti-RIg) coupled with fluorescein (Fl), all for 30 min at room temperature. The cells were viewed using (A) phase contrast, (B) rhodamine, and (C) fluorescein optics.

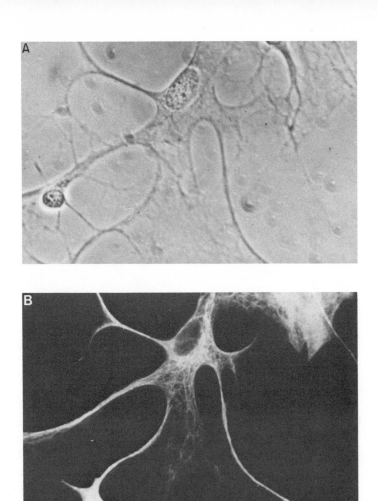

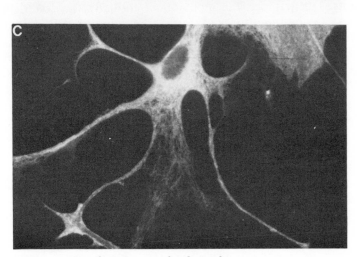

Figure 1 *(See facing page for legend.)*

GENERATION OF THE MONOCLONAL ANTIBODY

• C3H/He mice were immunized over the course of many months with a GFAP preparation from human postmortem spinal cord, which had been shown to produce high-titer, specific antisera to GFAP in rabbits (Pruss 1979). Spleen cells from mice with high serum titers were fused with NS1 cells. Hybridoma supernatants were screened by (1) a plate-binding assay using GFAP-coated wells and ultimately by (2) indirect immunofluorescence using acid-ethanol-fixed primary cultures from either fetal rat cerebrum or neonatal rat corpus callosum (the latter with more than 85% astrocytes). GFAP and most other intermediate filament classes, except neurofilament, are preserved in this fixation procedure. The antibody-secreting hybridoma described below was cloned three times.

THE MONOCLONAL ANTIBODY HISTOCHEMICALLY STAINS ALL CLASSES OF INTERMEDIATE FILAMENT

• When primary cell cultures from corpus callosum were stained with the monoclonal antibody, the intermediate filaments in the large, flat astrocytic cells were well labeled, whereas small, dark cells (presumably oligodendrocytes) were not. The same culture double-labeled with rabbit anti-GFAP gave a superimposable pattern (Fig. 1).

In the optic nerve culture, it was found that the monoclonal antibody labeled, in addition to the classical astrocytes defined by rabbit anti-GFAP sera, a population of flat cells that are largely derived from meninges and presumably contained the vimentin-type filaments. Furthermore, the monoclonal antibody was found to stain all types of cells in cultures of dorsal root ganglion (DRG), including fibroblasts (flat cells), Schwann cells (long bipolar cells), and neurons (Fig. 2).

In frozen sections of skeletal muscle, Z-lines were stained with the monoclonal antibody, raising the possibility that desmin is also recognized by this antibody (see the results of electrophoretic analysis below).

It is known that colchicine or Colcemid treatment of PtK_2 cells, which contain both vimentin-type and keratin-type filaments, causes the vimentin-type filaments to condense around the nucleus while leaving the keratin-type filaments spread over the cytoplasm (Osborn et al. 1980). Immunocytochemistry of colchicine-treated PtK_2 cells showed that both these filament systems are recognized by our monoclonal antibody (Fig. 3).

Pretreatment of cultured neural cells with rabbit anti-GFAP sera blocked the binding of the monoclonal antibody to astrocytes but not

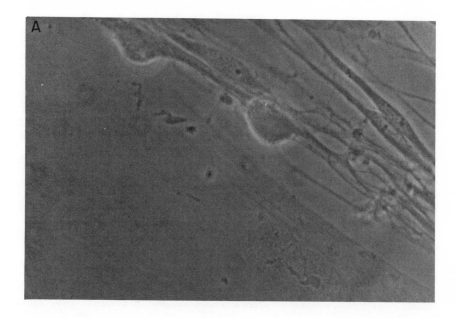

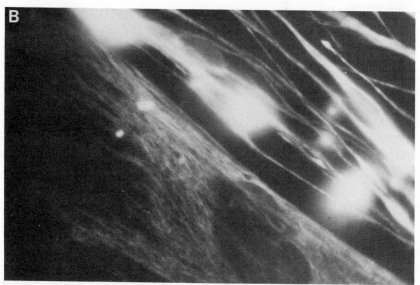

Figure 2
Labeling of rat DRG cultures with the monoclonal antibody. Cells were fixed
with acid ethanol and labeled with hybridoma supernatant overnight at 4°C
followed by goat anti–mouse immunoglobulin (G anti-MIg) coupled with
fluorescein (Fl). Cells were viewed using (A) phase contrast and (B) fluorescein optics.

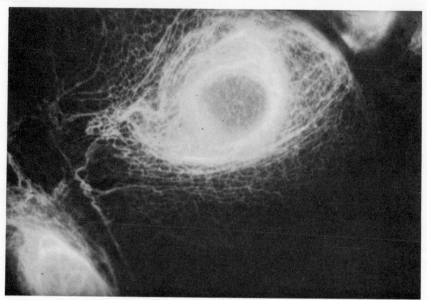

Figure 3
Effect of colchicine treatment on cultured PtK_2 cells. PtK_2 cells were treated with 10^{-5} M colchicine for 48 hr prior to fixation with acid ethanol. The cells were then incubated with hybridoma supernatant for 30 min at room temperature followed by G anti-MIg coupled with rhodamine (Rd). Cells were viewed using rhodamine optics.

to other cell types. Similarly, anti-vimentin sera blocked the binding of the monoclonal antibody to Schwann cells and fibroblasts in DRG cultures but not to neurons. It thus appears that the monoclonal antibody recognizes all five classes of intermediate filament (Table 1).

THE MONOCLONAL ANTIBODY STAINS THE ELECTROPHORETIC BANDS OF ALL CLASSES OF INTERMEDIATE FILAMENTS

• After SDS-polyacrylamide gel electrophoresis of either crude or purified filament preparations and subsequent treatment of the gels with our monoclonal antibody, the protein bands recognized by the antibody can be detected using a radioiodinated second antibody to mouse immunoglobulin followed by autoradiography (Burridge 1978).

When whole rat spinal cord was analyzed in this manner, the 200K, 145K, and 70K neurofilament subunits as well as the 58K vimentin and 50K GFAP were all labeled. In addition, the antibody labeled a band at 66K molecular weight (Fig. 4). Similar analysis of 3T3 and BHK cells as well as purified vimentin and desmin also showed that both of these intermediate filament subunits bind the monoclonal antibody. Keratin prepared from bovine hoof was similarly shown to be labeled by this antibody.

Analysis of the axoplasm prepared from squid and the marine worm, *Myxicola*, showed that the monoclonal antibody also recognizes a determinant present on both the neurofilament subunits of these invertebrates (a 200K and 60K doublet in squid and a 160K and 150K doublet in *Myxicola*) even though the molecular weights of the invertebrate subunits are very different from each other and from those of the vertebrate microfilaments. Thus, these electrophoretic analyses demonstrate that this monoclonal antibody recognizes a common and highly conserved domain shared by all five classes of intermediate filament, as well as a 66K protein present in every vertebrate and invertebrate filament preparation analyzed.

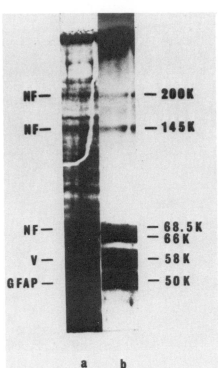

Figure 4

Immunoautoradiography of SDS-polyacrylamide gel prepared using proteins from whole rat spinal cord. Proteins were extracted from freshly dissected spinal cord by boiling in 2% SDS, 2% 2-mercaptoethanol in 0.1 M Tris (pH 6.8). Electrophoresis of the gels was performed and immunoautoradiography performed using a modification of the method of Burridge (1978). The Coomassie brilliant blue R staining pattern of the gel is seen in the left lane (a), and the autoradiograph of the same gel is seen in the right lane (b).

CONCLUSION

• A monoclonal antibody was obtained that specifically recognizes all five classes of intermediate filament by immunocytochemistry. Electrophoresis and immunoautoradiography using this antibody demonstrated that all intermediate filament subunit proteins share a common and highly conserved domain and that these filaments probably share a common subunit. This antibody should aid in histological and biochemical studies of intermediate filaments, including the search for new filament classes or proteins. In addition, this antibody will be a valuable probe of the interaction between intermediate filaments and other intracellular structures and may provide the means of specifically disrupting intermediate filament assembly as a way of determining its function.

REFERENCES

Burridge, K. 1978. Direct identification of specific glycoproteins and antigens in sodium dodecyl sulphate gels. *Methods Enzymol.* **50**:54.

Lazarides, E. 1980. Intermediate filaments as mechanical integrators of cellular space. *Nature* **283**:249.

Osborn, M., W.W. Franke, and K. Weber. 1980. Direct demonstration of the presence of two immunologically distinct intermediate-sized filament systems in the same cell by double immunofluorescence microscopy. *Exp. Cell Res.* **125**:37.

Pruss, R.M. 1979. Thy-1 antigen on astrocytes in long-term cultures of rat central nervous system. *Nature* **280**:688.

Raff, M.C., K.L. Fields, S. Hakomori, R. Mirsky, R.M. Pruss, and J. Winter. 1979. Studies on marker-identified rat glial and neuronal cells in culture: Antigens, bacterial toxin-binding properties and glycolipids. *Brain Res.* **174**:283.

An Immunochemical Approach to the Purification and Characterization of Glial Growth Factor

GREG LEMKE and JEREMY P. BROCKES

Division of Biology
California Institute of Technology
Pasadena, California 91125

• Recent advances in neural cell culture techniques have led to the definition of many "factors," usually soluble components that are extracted from tissue or released by cultured cells and that affect cellular differentiation or proliferation in vitro (Varon and Bunge 1978). These components are often present at low levels and their assay may be relatively time consuming. For these reasons, the purification of factors, upon which further progress depends, has proven very difficult. The derivation of monoclonal antibodies after immunization with partially purified fractions will clearly be a powerful tool in this field. An excellent example has been the recent derivation of a monoclonal antibody to human leukocyte interferon by Secher and Burke (1980).

Aside from their use in quantitation of the factors (e.g., radioimmunoassay) and for purification (e.g., affinity chromatography), such antibodies will be valuable in histochemical localization of these molecules in the nervous system and within cells. They may also prove useful as specific blocking agents in biological studies of the roles that such factors may play in vivo.

In this paper, we wish to summarize our research over the last three years on a new mitogenic component of the brain and pituitary and to describe the derivation of monoclonal antibodies to it.

GLIAL GROWTH FACTOR

• We have recently described the use of immunological methods both to identify and to purify rat Schwann cells from dissociated cultures of neonatal sciatic nerve (Brockes et al. 1977, 1979). These cultures contain only Schwann cells and fibroblasts, as determined by antigenic criteria, and the fibroblasts may be effectively removed by treatment with antiserum to the Thy-1 antigen followed by complement-dependent lysis (Brockes et al. 1979). In a conventional tissue-culture medium containing 10% fetal calf serum, the Schwann cells divide very slowly, taking 7–10 days to double in number. They are stimulated to divide by an activity present in extracts of the brain and pituitary (Brockes et al. 1979). The activity can be assayed by measuring the incorporation of [^{125}I]iododeoxyuridine (IUdR) into Schwann cells growing in microwells. Under optimal conditions, this incorporation is stimulated 30- to 100-fold.

Preliminary studies (Raff et al. 1978) with crude extracts have indicated that the activity is restricted in its distribution to the brain and pituitary, that it is labile to boiling and proteolytic digestion, and that it is apparently novel, since a variety of purified pituitary hormones and other mitogenic factors such as fibroblast growth factor (FGF) and epidermal growth factor (EGF) have no effect on Schwann cell proliferation. The activity in brain shows a 6- to 10-fold regional variation in specific activity (Brockes et al. 1981). One area, the caudate nucleus, yields extracts of an even higher specific activity

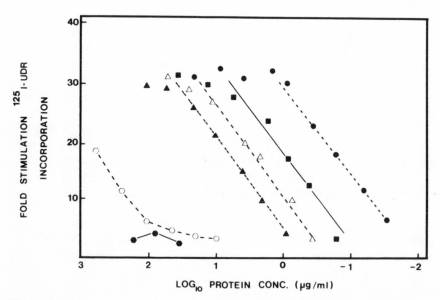

Figure 1
Dose response curves for various fractions in the GGF purification procedure. (●) Crude extract; (O) (NH$_4$)$_2$SO$_4$ fraction; (▲) CM-cellulose fraction; (△) AcA 44 gel filtration fraction; (■) second gel filtration fraction; (●) phospho-cellulose fraction.

than those of pituitary. The activities in the caudate and pituitary extracts are indistinguishable by chromatographic and electrophoretic criteria (Brockes and Lemke 1981). The regional variation suggests

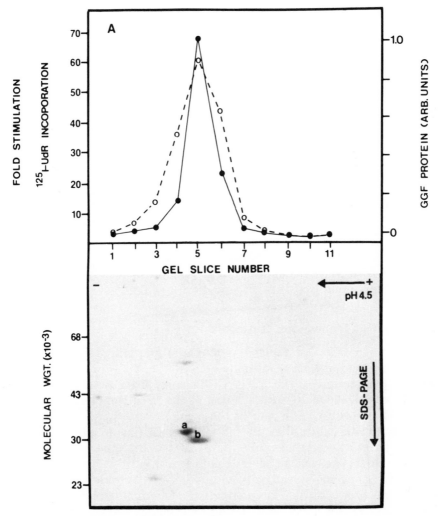

Figure 2
GGF activity on native gel electrophoresis of the most-purified fraction (*top*) and second dimension SDS electrophoresis of the native gel (*bottom*). Aliquots (5 μg) of the phosphocellulose fraction were run on parallel, small-scale, pH-4.5 polyacrylamide gels. One gel was sliced, eluted, and assayed in the Schwann cell proliferation assay. The other was laid on top of an SDS-polyacrylamide slab gel and analyzed by a second dimension of electrophoresis, followed by staining with Coomassie blue. The values of fold stimulation (o) have been converted to protein units (•) by using the logarithmic dose-response curves shown in Fig. 1. (Reprinted, with permission, from Brockes et al. 1980.)

that the factor, which had tentatively been named glial growth factor (GGF), is a component of nerve cells.

Partial Purification of GGF

The activity has been purified more than 4000-fold from a pool of 10 kg of frozen pituitaries and 4000 lyophilized anterior lobes, using the Schwann cell microwell proliferation assay (Brockes et al. 1980; Brockes and Lemke 1981) (Fig. 1). The most-purified (phosphocellulose) fraction is roughly 30% pure, but only 1.2 mg total protein was obtained from the preparation. The activity resides in a basic protein of m.w. ~6 $\times$ 10^4 that exists as a dimer of two subunits of m.w. 3 $\times$ 10^4, as determined by native and denaturing gel electrophoresis (Fig. 2). The mitogenic effect of the phosphocellulose fraction on cultured Schwann cells is illustrated in Figure 3.

The phosphocellulose fraction is also active on astrocytes in dissociated cultures of the rat corpus callosum, as evidenced by [^{3}H]thymidine autoradiography and immunofluorescent labeling, and on rat muscle fibroblasts (Brockes and Lemke 1981). These activities comigrate on native gel electrophoresis with the activity against Schwann cells. The phosphocellulose fraction is inactive on oligodendrocytes, microglia, and 3T3 cells.

Derivation of Monoclonal Antibodies to GGF

BALB/c mice were immunized with partially purified fractions of GGF. Each intraperitoneal injection consisted of 100–200 μg of total protein (containing 10–20 μg of GGF), complexed with 250 μg of poly(I):poly(C) as an adjuvant. On day 24 the mice were boosted with the same procedure. The sera of these mice were found to contain antibody to GGF, since they reacted with the GGF band after SDS gel electrophoresis and transfer onto diazotized paper (Renart et al. 1979; W. Lin and H. Kasamatsu, pers. comm.).

After fusing the spleen cells with NS1 cells, hybridoma supernatants were first screened for production of immunoglobulin with a solid-phase ELISA assay. Ig-secreting hybridomas were subsequently screened for anti-GGF production by an indirect immunoprecipitation assay modeled after that of Secher and Burke (1980). The supernatants were incubated with partially purified GGF, and after further incubation with carrier mouse IgG and rabbit anti–mouse IgG, immune complexes were removed by centrifugation. The supernatants were then assayed for residual GGF activity in the Schwann cell microwell proliferation assay (Fig. 4).

Sixteen positive clones have been derived from two fusions (71 Ig-secreting clones were obtained), and four have been characterized

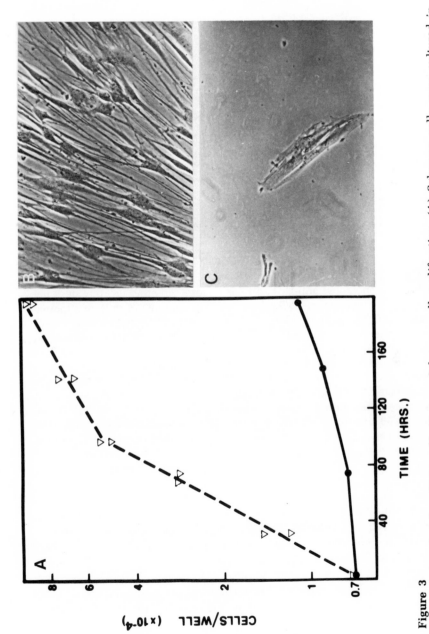

Figure 3
Effect of the phosphocellulose fraction on Schwann cell proliferation. (A) Schwann cells were cultured in medium with 10% fetal calf serum alone (●), or with 2 μg/ml phosphocellulose fraction (▽). (B) Phase-contrast photomicrograph of cells cultured for 5 days in the presence of GGF. (C) Cells cultured for 5 days in the absence of GGF.

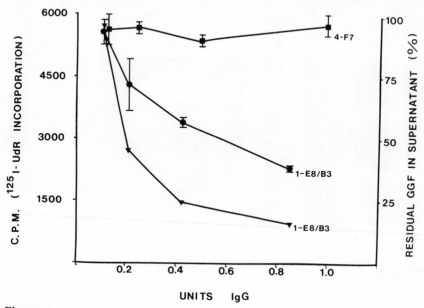

Figure 4

Titration of monoclonal anti-GGF. 4-F7 is a clone secreting IgG that does not react with GGF, whereas 1-E8/B3 does. Varying amounts of culture supernatant were incubated with the CM-cellulose fraction of GGF for 30 min at 37°C. Carrier mouse IgG and purified rabbit anti–mouse IgG were added and incubated overnight at 4°C. After centrifugation for 4 min at 20,000g, the supernatant was assayed for its ability to stimulate IUdR incorporation into Schwann cells in microwells (■ and ●). The decrease in stimulation by 1-E8/B3 is corrected by the logarithmic dosage relationship to give the amount of factor protein remaining in the supernatant (▼). One unit of IgG is the amount in 40 μl of 4-F7 culture supernatant as determined with a quantitative ELISA assay. The values for 1-E8/B3 are normalized to this. Each point is ±S.D. of three microwell assays.

in more detail. Each of these four secretes IgG, and each antibody appears to require indirect immunoprecipitation of immune complex in order to demonstrate clear inhibition in the proliferation assay. One-step incubations of the hybridoma supernatants with GGF solution proved to be ineffective, as shown in Figure 5 (cf. Secher and Burke 1980). These monoclonal antibodies may not, therefore, be directed against determinants that are important in stimulating Schwann cell proliferation.

We are currently investigating the utility of these reagents for affinity purification of GGF. They will also be important in projected studies on the localization of the molecule as well as in investigations of its possible role in nerve-stimulated mitosis and regeneration (Brockes and Lemke 1981).

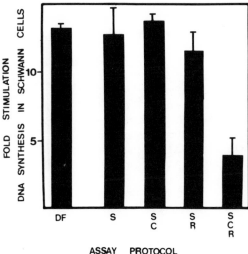

Figure 5
Inhibition requires indirect immunoprecipitation. Various combinations of immunore-agents and GGF solution (CM-cellulose fraction) were tested in the two-step incubation and assay procedure described in Fig. 4. (DF) First step is 10 μl of GGF solution with 20 μl Dulbecco's modified Eagle's medium plus 10% fetal calf serum (DFCS); second (overnight) step is 12 μl of DFCS. (S) First step is 10 μl of GGF solution with 20 μl of 1-E8/B3 anti-GGF hybridoma supernatant; second step is 12 μl DFCS. (SC) First step is as in S; second step is 7 μl of normal mouse IgG solution and 5 μl of DFCS. (SR) First step is as in S; second step is 5 μl of a rabbit anti–mouse IgG solution and 7 μl of DFCS. (SCR) First step is as in S; second step is 7 μl of normal mouse IgG solution and 5 μl of rabbit anti–mouse IgG solution. In other controls, carrier (normal) mouse IgG and rabbit anti–mouse IgG were found to give no inhibition in the absence of hybridoma supernatant. Therefore, only with supernatant, followed by anti–mouse IgG and carrier mouse IgG (to ensure equivalence), is there significant precipitation of GGF activity.

ACKNOWLEDGMENT

• This work was supported by a grant to J.P.B. from the Kroc Foundation.

REFERENCES

Brockes, J.P. and G.E. Lemke. 1981. The neuron as a source of mitogen. *Soc. Dev. Biol. Symp.* **V:** (in press).

Brockes, J.P., K.L. Fields, and M.C. Raff. 1977. A surface antigenic marker for rat Schwann cells. *Nature* **266:**364.

————. 1979. Studies on cultured rat Schwann cells. I. Establishment of purified populations from peripheral nerve. *Brain Res.* **165:**105.

Brockes, J.P., K. Fryxell, and G.E. Lemke. 1981. Studies on cultured Schwann cells—The induction of myelin synthesis, and the control of their proliferation by a new growth factor. In *Glial-neurone interactions* (ed. J.E. Treherne). Cambridge University Press, Cambridge, England. (In press.)

Brockes, J.P., G.E. Lemke, and D.R. Balzer, Jr. 1980. Purification and preliminary characterization of a glial growth factor from the bovine pituitary. *J. Biol. Chem.* **255:**8374.

Raff, M.C., E. Abney, J.P. Brockes, and A. Hornby-Smith. 1978. Schwann cell growth factors. *Cell* **15:**813.

Renart, J., J. Reiser, and G. Stark. 1979. Transfer of proteins from gels to diazobenzyloxymethyl paper and detection with antisera. *Proc. Natl. Acad. Sci.* **76:**3116.

Secher, D.S. and D.C. Burke. 1980. A monoclonal antibody for the large-scale purification of human leukocyte interferon. *Nature* **285:**446.

Varon, S. and R. Bunge. 1978. Trophic mechanisms in the peripheral nervous system. *Annu. Rev. Neurosci.* **1:**327.

Monoclonal Antibodies as Probes for Ligand-Receptor Interactions: Studies of the Thyrotropin Receptor

EPHRAIM YAVIN,* ZIVA YAVIN, and
LEONARD D. KOHN

Section of Biochemistry of Cell Regulation
Laboratory of Biochemical Pharmacology
National Institute of Arthritis, Metabolism, and Digestive Diseases
National Institutes of Health
Bethesda, Maryland 20205

MICHAEL D. SCHNEIDER

Laboratory of Biochemical Genetics
National Heart, Lung, and Blood Institute
National Institutes of Health
Bethesda, Maryland 20205

• The receptor for thyrotropin (thyroid-stimulating hormone, or TSH) is the subject of enormous interest and controversy.

1. The subunit structure of the TSH receptor (Kohn 1978; Kohn et al. 1980, 1981) may comprise both a glycoprotein (as the primary high-affinity binding site) and a ganglioside, which discriminates among ligands that compete with TSH for binding and also induces a conformational change in the peptide hormone necessary for signal transduction by facilitating entry of TSH into the lipid bilayer to enable activation of the TSH-dependent adenylate cyclase.

2. Two ligands that compete for the TSH receptor are tetanus toxin (with similar ganglioside specificity for GD_{1b} and GT_1) and cholera toxin (with specificity, instead, for GM_1) (Mirsky et al. 1978; Raff et al. 1979). These toxins are also important cell markers and have dramatic physiological consequences.

3. Neural model systems that possess a receptor for TSH, functionally coupled to adenylate cyclase, include the embryonic chick retina (L.D. Kohn et al., unpubl.).

---

*On leave from the Department of Neurobiology, the Weizmann Institute of Science, Rehovot, Israel.

4. In myasthenia gravis, abnormal ligand-receptor interactions are attributable to autoantibodies against the nicotinic acetylcholine receptor; analogously, in Graves' disease, autoantibodies specifically bind the receptor for TSH (Smith and Hall 1974; Manley et al. 1974; Mukhtar et al. 1975; Mehdi and Nussey 1975; McKenzie and Zakarija 1977; Fenzi et al. 1978; McKenzie et al. 1978). However, this immunoglobulin fraction not only blocks the binding of TSH, but also functions itself as a potent hormone agonist, activating the TSH-dependent adenylate cyclase and concomitant thyroid function with a time course that is prolonged compared with that of the peptide hormone.

Structure-function relationships of the TSH receptor are amenable to study by monoclonal antibodies (Köhler and Milstein 1975) that resolve single-receptor determinants. Particular emphasis is placed on the question of whether, in the polyclonal immune response of Graves' disease, separate distinguishable epitopes or antibody populations are responsible, respectively, for inhibiting TSH binding and for long-acting thyroid stimulation.

PRODUCTION AND SCREENING OF HYBRIDOMA ANTIBODIES

• Three-month-old BALB/c mice were immunized subcutaneously with lithium-diiodosalicylate (LIS)-solubilized bovine thyroid membranes (Yavin et al. 1981), and their spleen cells were fused with P3-NS1/1-Ag4-1 mouse myeloma cells by standard techniques (Galfre et al. 1977; Trisler et al. 1981). Initial hybridoma colonies were assayed for antibody binding to thyroid membranes in suspension (400 μg protein/well) in the absence or presence of 1 x 10^{-6} M TSH by means of an indirect radioimmunoassay. In subsequent experiments, thyroid membranes were immobilized by adsorption to microtiter plates pretreated for 1 hour with 20 μg/ml of poly-L-lysine and assayed for binding of either hybridoma antibodies or radioiodinated TSH (E. Yavin et al., in prep.).

TSH INHIBITS BINDING OF SIX HYBRIDOMA ANTIBODIES

• Hybridoma colonies grew in 346 of 2268 wells seeded after two separate fusions, of which 55 synthesized antibody reactive with bovine thyroid membranes. These, in turn, were analyzed for antireceptor specificity by performing antibody incubation in the presence of unlabeled TSH or cholera toxin (1 x 10^{-6} M) (Table 1) and have been divided into five groups:

Table 1
Effects of Unlabelled TSH and Cholera Toxin on Monoclonal Antibody Binding to Bovine Thyroid Membranes, Detected by ^{125}I-labeled F(ab')$_2$ Binding

Group	Representative hybridoma clone	Unlabeled ligand added (1×10^{-6} M) (% of control binding in the absence of unlabelled ligand)	
		TSH	cholera toxin
I	T-18A3	100	94
II	T-21D10	0	50
III	T-28E4	20	10
IV	T-25E2	80	0
V	T-17D8	150	220

1. The binding of 46 anti-thyroid antibodies is unaffected by either ligand.
2. The binding of 5 hybridoma antibodies to thyroid membranes is completely blocked by unlabeled TSH but less than 50% inhibited by cholera toxin (Fig. 1).
3. One hybridoma antibody is inhibited 80% by TSH and 90% by cholera toxin.
4. One hybridoma antibody is completely blocked by cholera toxin alone.
5. The binding of two hybridoma antibodies, at the ligand concentration employed, is stimulated by both TSH (150% of control) and cholera toxin (200% of control).

No influence is detected using comparable concentrations of the

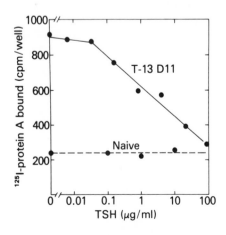

Figure 1
Unlabeled TSH inhibits hybridoma antibody (clone T-13D11) binding to immobilized bovine thyroid membranes, as determined by ^{125}I-labeled staphylococcal protein-A binding. Nonspecific ^{125}I-labeled protein-A binding was measured in the presence of the equivalent protein concentration of an antibody unreactive with thyroid membranes.

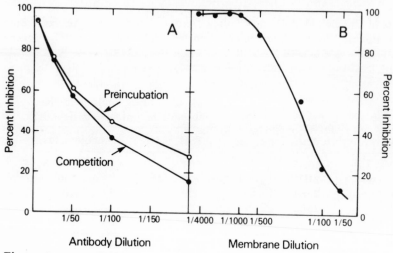

Figure 2

Monoclonal antibody (clone T-11E8) inhibits ^{125}I-labeled TSH binding to immobilized bovine thyroid membranes. (A) Effect of varying antibody concentration (45% ammonium sulfate precipitate from ascites fluid). Membranes were pretreated with antibody (o) or exposed to antibody and ^{125}I-labeled TSH concomitantly (•). (B) Effect of varying membrane concentration.

peptide hormones insulin or human chorionic gonadotropin (HCG); HCG was previously shown to bind the glycoprotein component of the TSH receptor but does not result in signal propagation.

Conversely, group-II antibodies (the ammonium sulfate precipi-

Table 2

Inhibition of ^{125}I-labeled TSH Binding by Ammonium Sulfate Preparations Derived from Ascites Fluid or Conditioned Medium of Hybridoma Clones Whose Antibody Binding Was Blocked by TSH

Hybridoma clone	Ascites (% inhibition)	Culture medium (% inhibition)
T-13D11	94	92
T-22A6	78	72
T-11E8	78	81
T-21D10	58	59
T-29C7	33	38

Ammonium sulfate fractions containing immunoglobulin from hybridoma-conditioned medium or ascites fluid were dialyzed and added at 0.1 mg/ml concomitantly with ^{125}I-labeled TSH. Results shown are corrected for ^{125}I-labeled TSH binding in the presence of an equal concentration of an anti−thyroid hybridoma antibody that was not inhibited by 1×10^{-6} M unlabeled TSH (group I, Table 1).

tates of hybridoma culture supernatants or ascites fluids) are inhibitors of ^{125}I-labeled TSH binding to thyroid membranes, either as pretreatment or when added concomitantly (Fig. 2; Table 2). The interaction of TSH and hybridoma antibodies is shown to be competitive in a double-reciprocal plot of assays performed at two concentrations of hybridoma antibody and multiple concentrations of TSH (Fig. 3).

Tetanus toxin, at 1×10^{-6} M, is a potent inhibitor of two of the group-II hybridoma antibodies blocked by TSH and, hence, discriminates among the set of antibodies that are candidates for probes against the receptor. Whether these differences in binding are a consequence of different affinities or different epitopes has not yet been determined.

MODULATION OF RECEPTOR-ANTIBODY INTERACTIONS BY CONCANAVALIN A

• The α-methyl-mannoside-binding plant lectin concanavalin A (Con A) (Sharon and Lis 1972) was previously shown to enhance ^{125}I-labeled TSH binding to bovine thyroid membranes or to liposomes containing the glycoprotein component of the TSH receptor (D. Tombaccini et al., in prep.). This interaction was not due to the formation of a complex between the lectin and hormone, required tetrameric Con A, and was ligand-specific (not associated with a measurable increase in the binding of ^{125}I-labeled cholera toxin). Among cell-surface events induced by tetrameric Con A is perturbation of mem-

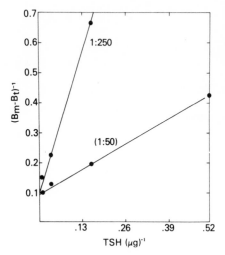

Figure 3
TSH inhibition of monoclonal antibody (T-13D11) binding is competitive, as demonstrated by a double-reciprocal plot of ^{125}I-labeled protein-A binding at 40 μg/ml (1:250) or 200 μg/ml (1:50) of antibody and varying concentrations of unlabeled TSH. Values on the abscissa are the reciprocal of maximal ^{125}I-labeled protein A bound (in the absence of TSH) minus the percentage of maximal ^{125}I-labeled protein A bound at each TSH concentration. Identical results were obtained with hybridoma T-11E8 antibody preparations; other group-II (Table 1) clones were not similarly tested.

brane fluidity. Earlier experiments involving TSH receptor components in liposomes similarly showed that substitutions in the phospholipid matrix that alter membrane fluidity (substitution of dioleoyl phosphatidylcholine for dipalmitoyl phosphatidylcholine) increase the binding of TSH but not tetanus toxin (Lee et al. 1978).

Accordingly, hybridoma antibody inhibition of ^{125}I-labeled TSH was studied under conditions of Con-A treatment that modulate TSH receptor expression (Fig. 4). Concomitant with increased ^{125}I-labeled TSH binding activity, antibody effectiveness as an inhibitor decreases. In preliminary experiments involving a library of monoclonal antibodies against human (Graves' disease) thyroid membranes, Con A is also shown to increase the binding of hybridoma antibodies specifically reacting with the TSH binding site (data not shown).

Three different TSH receptor preparations are capable of demonstrating both hybridoma antibody inhibition of TSH binding and Con-

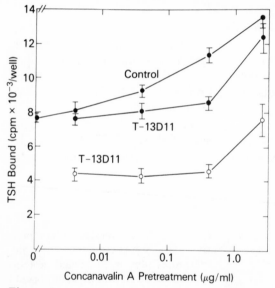

Figure 4

Con A modulates antibody-dependent inhibition of ^{125}I-labeled protein-A binding. Immobilized bovine thyroid membranes were pretreated with Con A at the concentrations noted, washed, then treated with antibody T-13D11 at (●) 11 μg/ml or (○) 111 μg/ml prior to incubation with ^{125}I-labeled TSH in the presence of 0.1 M α-methyl-mannoside to ensure that radioligand binding was not due to membrane-associated Con A. Results were analogous with all group-II antibodies.

A enhancement of TSH binding (Table 3): (1) immobilized thyroid membranes from patients with Graves' disease; (2) the immobilized glycoprotein component of TSH receptor (LIS-solubilized bovine thyroid membranes); or (3) liposomes containing the glycoprotein component of the receptor. Liposomes containing, instead, mixed bovine brain gangliosides, specifically bind ^{125}I-labeled TSH but show no modulation by Con A and no inhibition by the hybridoma antibodies. These results suggest that the hybridoma antibodies are against the glycoprotein component of the TSH receptor.

ANTIBODY BINDING TO RAT THYROID CELL LINES

• The hybridoma antibodies were also assayed against functional (FRT$_L$) and nonfunctional (FRT) clonal rat thyroid cell lines, obtained from F.S. Ambesi-Impiombato and H. G. Coon (Fig. 5). FRT$_L$ cells bind TSH and activate adenylate cyclase, responding physiologically with iodine uptake and production of thyroglobulin and thyroid hormone (Ambesi-Impiombato et al. 1980); FRT cells bind less than 20% as

Table 3
Effect of Monoclonal Antibody on ^{125}I-labeled TSH Binding to Human Thyroid Membranes, the Glycoprotein Component of the Bovine TSH Receptor, or Gangliosides

	TSH receptor preparation (^{125}I-labeled TSH bound, cpm [10^{-3}] per well)			
	Human (Graves' disease) thyroid membranes[1]	LIS-solubilized bovine thyroid membranes (glycoprotein component of TSH receptor)		Bovine brain gangliosides in liposomes[2]
		free[1]	in liposomes[2]	
Control	10.0	3.1	15.2	18.0
+ Con A	15.2	9.9	25.4	18.0
+ T-11E8	1.9	1.0	3.1	17.5

[1]Human thyroid membranes (5 μg) or LIS-solubilized bovine thyroid membranes (4 μg) were allowed to adsorb to poly-L-lysine-treated microtiter wells as described. Con-A pretreatment (20 μg/ml) was for 1 hr at 4°C in 20 mM Tris-acetate (pH 7.0). Treated membranes were washed twice, followed by addition of ^{125}I-labeled TSH (55,000 cpm/well). T-11E8 antibody (ammonium sulfate preparation of ascites fluid) was used at 10−12 μg/ml, added concomitantly with ^{125}I-labeled TSH.

[2]Assays using receptor components incorporated into liposomes employed a previously described filtration assay for ^{125}I-labeled TSH binding (Aloj et al. 1979) and incubation conditions detailed above.

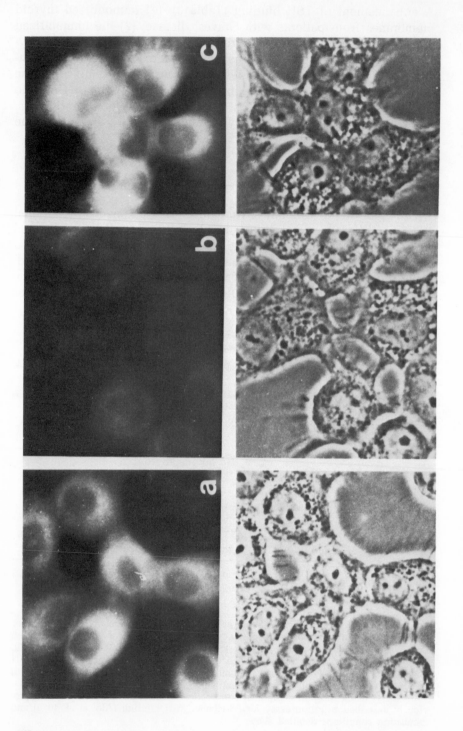

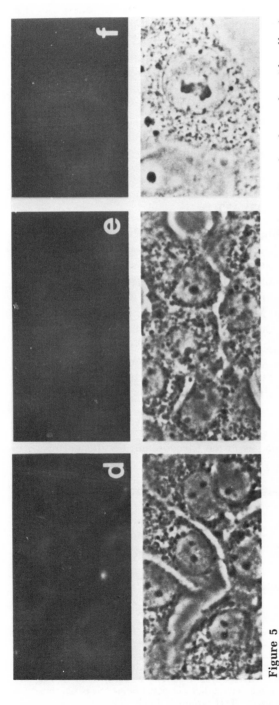

Figure 5
Anti-TSH receptor antibodies T-11E8 (*a,b,f*) and T-13D11 (*c,d*) label functional (FRT$_L$) clonal rat thyroid cells (*a* through e) but not nonfunctional (FRT) cells (*f*). Cells cultured on poly-L-lysine-treated glass coverslips for 3–4 days were fixed with 0.1% glutaraldehyde for 30 min, washed, and treated with 50 μg/ml of monoclonal antibody in the absence (*a,c,e,f*) or presence (*b,d*) of 1 mg/ml of TSH. A fluorescein-conjugated goat anti–mouse IgG was employed at 1:20 concentration. Functional cells incubated with a control antibody preparation are shown in e. Phase-contrast microscopy of each field is shown for comparison. Comparable results were obtained with unfixed cells at 4°C.

much TSH and are unresponsive (F. S. Ambesi-Impiombato and H. G. Coon, in prep.). By indirect immunofluorescence, those antibodies thought to recognize the glycoprotein component of the receptor label FRT$_L$ but not FRT cells and are blocked by TSH (1 mg/ml). As the solubilized membranes of FRT cells had been shown to contain less than 50% of TSH binding sites obtained with FRT$_L$ cells, the differences between the clonal cell lines or between their membranes may be due to defects in receptor expression such as processing and insertion into the surface membrane. Monoclonal antibodies may be valuable probes for investigating receptor biosynthesis, regulation, and expression in normal and abnormal cells.

STUDIES OF THYROID ACTIVATION

• Even at 10- to 100-fold higher concentrations than used to inhibit TSH binding completely, none of the monoclonal antibodies was able to activate the TSH-dependent adenylate cyclase (Salomon 1979) when either thyroid membrane preparations (Table 4) or thyroid membrane slices were employed (E. Yavin et al., unpubl., in collaboration with J. McKenzie and M. Zakarija). The inability of monoclonal antibodies directed primarily at the glycoprotein component of the TSH receptor to stimulate the adenylate cyclase system is consistent with the proposal that the glycoprotein component is itself insufficient for TSH signal transduction and that receptor-activation coupling may require the additional participation of the ganglioside.

Table 4
Inability of Monoclonal Antibodies to the Glycoprotein Component of TSH Receptor to Stimulate Adenylate Cyclase Activity in Bovine Thyroid Membranes

Assay addition	Adenylate cyclase activity (pmoles cAMP per 15 min per mg membrane protein)
Basal control	106
+ TSH (1 × 10^{-7} M)	388
+ T-18A3 (control antibody)	110
+ T-13D11	105
+ T-21D10	99
+ T-22A6	110
+ T-11E8	104

Antisera were tested as ammonium sulfate fractions of culture media at 1–1.2 mg/ml for results shown. No effect on adenylate cyclase activity was seen at 10–120 μg/ml as well. T-18A3 control antibody binds bovine thyroid membranes but is not measurably inhibited by 1 × 10^{-6} M unlabeled TSH (group I, Table 1).

Current experiments are attempting to identify monoclonal antibodies that are cyclase activators and to establish whether they bind a receptor complex comprising both glycoprotein and ganglioside or even are directed at the ganglioside alone.

DISCUSSION

• Monoclonal antibodies were obtained whose binding to thyroid membrane preparations is specifically and competitively inhibited by TSH. The antibodies react with bovine thyroid membranes, human thyroid membranes (from patients with Graves' disease), and functional but not nonfunctional clonal rat thyroid cell lines. The antibodies block ^{125}I-labeled TSH binding to liposomes containing the solubilized glycoprotein component of the receptor and are unable to inhibit TSH binding to liposomes containing ganglioside. The observed interaction with the glycoprotein component is insufficient to activate the TSH-dependent adenylate cyclase. Because they discriminate among other ligands that compete for the TSH receptor, the antibodies may be useful to map a partially shared repertoire of receptor antigenic domains. The antibodies may be employed, as well, to elucidate the molecular mechanisms that underlie receptor modulation and expression. Finally, these techniques and approaches should provide a means to resolve the nature of Graves' disease autoantibodies, the specific determinant to which they bind, and the mechanisms of receptor-activation coupling by which hyperthyroidism occurs.

REFERENCES

Aloj, S.M., G. Lee, E.F. Grollman, F. Beguinot, E. Consiglio, and L.D. Kohn. 1979. Role of phospholipids in the structure and function of the thyrotropin receptor. J. Biol. Chem. **254:**9040.

Ambesi-Impiombato, F.S., L.A.M. Parks, and H.G. Coon. 1980. Culture of hormone-dependent functional epithelial cells from rat thyroids. Proc. Natl. Acad. Sci. **77:**3455.

Fenzi, G., E. Macchia, L. Bartalena, F. Mazzanti, L. Baschieri, and L.J. De Groot. 1978. Radioreceptor assay for TSH: Its use to detect thyroid-stimulating immunoglobulins. J. Endocrinol. Invest. **1:**17.

Galfre, G., S.C. Howe, C. Milstein, G.W. Butcher, and J.G. Howard. 1977. Antibodies to major histocompatibility antigens produced by hybrid cell lines. Nature **266:**550.

Köhler, G. and C. Milstein, 1975. Continuous cultures of fused cells secreting antibody of predefined specificity. Nature **256:**495.

Kohn, L.D. 1978. Relationships, structure, and function of receptors for glycoprotein hormones, bacterial toxins, and interferon. In Receptors and recognition (ed. P. Cuatracasas and M.F. Greaves), vol. 5, p. 134. Chapman and Hall, London.

Kohn, L.D., E. Consiglio, M.J.S. De Wolf, E.F. Grollman, F.D. Ledley, G. Lee, and N.P. Morris. 1980. Thyrotropin receptors and gangliosides. *Adv. Exp. Med. Biol.* **125**:487.

Kohn, L.D., E. Consiglio, S.M. Aloj, F. Beguinot, M.J.S. De Wolf, E. Yavin, Z. Yavin, M.F. Meldolesi, S. Shifrin, D.L. Gill, P. Vitti, G. Lee, W.A. Valente, and E.F. Grollman. 1981. The structure of the thyrotropin (TSH) receptor: Potential role of gangliosides and relationship to receptors for interferon and bacterial toxins. In *International cell biology 1980–1981* (ed. H.G. Schweiger), p. 696. Lange and Springer, Berlin, Federal Republic of Germany.

Lee, G., E. Consiglio, W. Habig, S. Dyer, M.C. Hardegree, and L.D. Kohn. 1978. Structure:function studies of receptors for thyrotropin and tetanus toxin: Lipid modulation of effector binding to the glycoprotein receptor component. *Biochem. Biophys. Res. Commun.* **83**:313.

Manley, S.W., J.R. Bourke, and R.W. Hawkes. 1974. The thyrotropin receptor in guinea pig thyroid homogenate: General properties. *J. Endocrinol.* **61**:437.

McKenzie, J.M. and M. Zakarija. 1977. LATS in Graves' disease. *Recent Prog. Horm. Res.* **33**:29.

McKenzie, J.M., M. Zakarija, and A. Sato. 1978. Reconsideration of thyroid-stimulating immunoglobulins as the cause of hyperthyroidism in Graves' disease. *J. Clin. Endocrinol. Metab.* **7**:31.

Mehdi, S.W. and S.S. Nussey. 1975. A radio ligand receptor assay for the long-acting thyroid stimulator. Inhibition by the long-acting thyroid stimulator of the binding of radioiodinated thyroid-stimulating hormone to human thyroid membranes. *Biochem. J.* **145**:105.

Mirsky, R., L.M.B. Wendon, P. Black, C. Stolkin, and D. Bray. 1978. Tetanus toxin: A cell surface marker for neurons in culture. *Brain Res.* **148**:251.

Mukhtar, E.D., B.R. Smith, G.A. Pyle, R. Hall, and P. Vice. 1975. Relation of thyroid-stimulating immunoglobulins to thyroid function and effects of surgery, radioiodine, and antithyroid drugs. *Lancet* **1**:713.

Raff, M.C., K.L. Fields, S.-I. Hakomori, R. Mirsky, R.M. Pruss, and J. Winter. 1979. Cell-type specific markers for distinguishing and studying neurons and the major classes of glial cells in culture. *Brain Res.* **174**:283.

Salomon, Y. 1979. Adenylate cyclase. *Adv. Cyclic Nucleotide Res.* **10**:35.

Sharon, N. and H. Lis. 1972. Lectins: Cell-agglutinating and sugar-specific proteins. *Science* **177**:949.

Smith, B.R. and R. Hall. 1974. Binding of thyroid stimulators to thyroid membranes. *FEBS Lett.* **42**:301.

Trisler, G.D., M.D. Schneider, and M. Nirenberg. 1981. A topographic gradient of molecules in avian retina can be used to determine neuron position. *Proc. Natl. Acad. Sci.* **78**:2145.

Yavin, E., Z. Yavin, M.D. Schneider, and L.D. Kohn. 1981. Monoclonal antibodies to the thyrotropin receptor: Implications for receptor structure and the action of autoantibodies in Graves' disease. *Proc. Natl. Acad. Sci.* **78**:3180.

Antibodies to Pure Cholinergic Synaptic Vesicles, Nerve Terminals, and Their Plasma Membranes

REGIS B. KELLY, STEVEN S. CARLSON,
RANDALL J. VON WEDEL, JOAN E. HOOPER,
GEORGE P. MILJANICH, and ALLAN R.
BRASIER
Department of Biochemistry and Biophysics
University of California
San Francisco, California 94143

• We are interested in the molecular events that occur during transmitter release from nerve terminals. It is known that release is triggered by the entry of calcium through voltage-sensitive calcium channels. The elevation of intraterminal calcium causes the synaptic vesicle, a spherical organelle packed with neurotransmitter, to fuse to the presynaptic plasma membrane at morphologically specialized sites called active zones. The membrane components of the synaptic vesicle thus are thought to be recovered by an adsorptive pinocytosis route involving coated vesicles. We are particularly interested in the recognition events between vesicle and active zone as well as the mechanism of membrane recycling.

Our initial approach was to purify synaptic vesicles to as close to biochemical homogeneity as possible and to use them to generate conventional antibodies. If an antiserum unique to vesicle antigens could be generated, then it could be used to isolate presynaptic plasma membranes. A simple purification procedure for presynaptic plasma membranes would be an important tool in our studies.

The cholinergic vesicles of the electric organ of the marine ray *Narcine brasiliensis* were chosen for study because of their availability in relatively abundant amounts and because of the convenient vesicle marker, acetylcholine (ACh), that is used to trace the vesicles during their purification. The purified vesicles have a ratio of ACh to protein several hundred–fold higher than that of the starting material (Carlson et al. 1978).

The synaptic vesicle of N. *brasiliensis* has been characterized (Wagner et al. 1978). It contains a high concentration of ACh (520 mM), ATP, and GTP but no soluble intravesicular proteins. Isolated intact vesicles have eight major polypeptides, as shown by SDS-acrylamide gel electrophoresis. Six of these are unique to the vesicle. Five of these unique polypeptides are exposed on the cytoplasmic side of the vesicle, whereas the sixth, a 33-kD insoluble protein, is largely located on the inner surface (Wagner and Kelly 1979). The bulk nonlipid component, however, did not enter the gel during electrophoresis. This 100–300-kD material is assumed to be a proteoglycan since it contains both carbohydrate and protein. When SDS gels of vesicle proteins are exposed to radioactive wheat germ agglutinin (WGA), binding is observed to this putative glucosamineglycan material and also to the six peptides unique to synaptic vesicles. Intact iodinated synaptic vesicles do not bind to WGA beads (Fig. 1). After lysis by sonication, extensive binding is observed. The presence of N-acetylglucosamine in excess amounts inhibits the binding. We conclude that the majority of the carbohydrate groups are inside the synaptic vesicle. Since the five unique peptides from the cytoplasmic surface are readily labeled by membrane-impermeable reagents and have WGA-binding sites on the interior of the vesicle, we conclude that they are transmembrane proteins.

MOST OF THE ANTIBODIES IN THE SERUM SPECIFICALLY BIND TO SYNAPTIC VESICLES

• Rabbits were immunized with the purified synaptic vesicles in complete Freund's adjuvant, either with or without sonication. The fraction of antibodies that is specific to the synaptic vesicle was determined by adsorbing the antiserum against a sonicated electric-organ-membrane fraction of N. *brasiliensis* that is essentially free of synaptic vesicles and then measuring the residual titer. Approximately 60% of the antibody titer are removed by adsorption. As a control, adsorption of the serum with sonicated synaptic vesicles removed 96% of the antibody titer. The implication of these results is that roughly one-half of the antibodies produced are specific for synaptic vesicles. This adsorbed serum can apparently be used as a specific probe for synaptic vesicles, as shown below.

THE PRESENCE OF SYNAPTIC VESICLES CAN BE QUANTITATED BY A SPECIFIC RADIOIMMUNOASSAY

• An indirect radioimmunoassay (RIA) was set up to assay quantitatively for synaptic vesicle antigens (Fig. 2). This RIA utilizes ^{125}I-radiolabeled synaptic vesicle antigen, the polyclonal serum, and

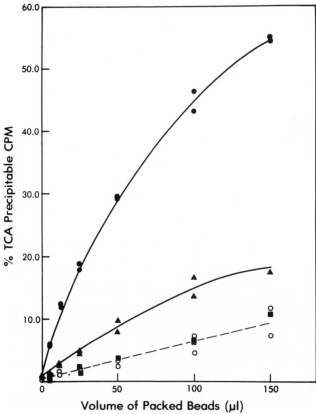

Figure 1

Precipitation of whole vesicles with WGA beads. Intact synaptic vesicles were labeled with ^{125}I-labeled diazotized iodosulfonilic acid. An aliquot of ^{125}I-labeled synaptic vesicles was sonicated so that it completely released its contents. Sonicated ^{125}I-labeled synaptic vesicles were incubated with WGA–Sepharose CL-4B beads in the presence (o) and absence (●) of 150 mg/ml N-acetylglucosamine. Whole vesicles were incubated under the same conditions with (■) and without (▲) N-acetylglucosamine. After an overnight incubation, the beads were pelleted, washed several times, and counted.

Staphylococcus aureus cells for the precipitation of antibody-antigen complexes. The assay can be shown in the following way to be both specific for synaptic membrane antigens and sensitive (Carlson and Kelly 1980):

1. ACh cosediments with the material detected by RIA on both

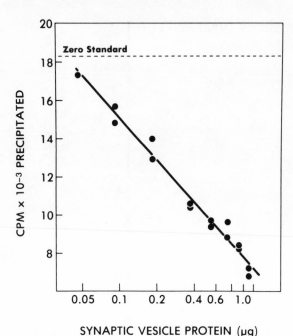

SYNAPTIC VESICLE PROTEIN (µg)

Figure 2
A standard curve for the RIA. The iodinated
synaptic vesicle antigen precipitated by antiserum and S. *aureus* is plotted against the
amount of unlabeled synaptic vesicle protein
added to the reaction mixture. The zero control
(no unlabeled vesicle antigen added) is shown
by the dotted line.

    glycerol and sucrose density gradients. The ratio of ACh
concentration to antigenicity, as determined by the RIA, is
constant in all the fractions of the glycerol gradient and is
close to that observed for vesicles purified to homogeneity.

2. Another demonstration of the specificity of the immunoad-
sorbed polyclonal serum is that during purification of the
vesicles, the antigen and ACh copurify with a constant ACh
concentration/antigenicity ratio at all steps of the procedure.

3. An indication of the sensitivity of the serum to synaptic
vesicles is that even though the vesicles make up only about
0.5% of the material in the original homogenate, the ratio of
ACh concentration to antigenicity could still be measured
and is indistinguishable from that found with pure vesicles.

THE ANTIBODY RECOGNIZES DIFFERENT
TYPES OF NERVE TERMINALS

• The polyclonal serum cross-reacts very nicely with the mammalian central and peripheral nervous systems. It binds selectively to nerve terminals and not to axons or to cell bodies. For instance, using a double-fluorescence-labeling technique in which the neuromuscular juntion (NMJ) is identified by the binding of rhodamine-conjugated α-bungarotoxin and the antibody-antigen binding of a fluorescein-conjugated goat anti–rabbit IgG antibody, Sanes and colleagues (Sanes et al. 1979) have shown that the nerve terminals at the NMJ of mammalian, amphibian, and avian skeletal muscle bind the polyclonal antiserum. Hooper and colleagues (Hooper et al. 1980) have expanded the list of tissues examined for binding of the serum, using indirect staining techniques (peroxidase-antiperoxidase and immunofluorescence). Shared antigenic determinants are found in (1) cholinergic terminals (NMJ, sympathetic ganglion, parasympathetic postganglionic terminals, synaptic areas of the hippocampus and cerebellum) and (2) some, but not all, noncholinergic terminals (the adrenal sympathetic postganglionic terminals, peptidergic terminals in the neurohypophysis, and adrenal chromaffin cells are labeled). However, the molecular layer of the cerebellum and those laminae of the dentate gyrus that receive hippocampal association and commissural input do not bind the antibodies.

This demonstration of shared antigens among different types of mammalian nerve terminals and fish synaptic vesicles supports the idea that these determinants are evolutionarily conserved. In addition, a relationship seems to exist among different neurotransmitter types of mammalian nerve terminals previously thought to be unrelated.

THE ANTIGEN IS PRESENT INSIDE SYNAPTIC VESICLES

• A group of three experiments was performed to localize the antigens in the nerve terminal (von Wedel et al. 1981).

1. Transverse cryostat sections of an unstimulated frog cutaneous pectoris fiber, labeled with fluorescein-conjugated goat anti–rabbit IgG reveal specific antibody binding in the region of the NMJ (Fig. 3A).
2. In whole mounts of unstimulated cutaneous pectoris fibers, no antibody binding in the region of the NMJ is observed (Fig. 3B,C). This lack of binding cannot be explained by the inability of the antibody to permeate into the nerve terminal, since extensive binding is observed after treatment with β-

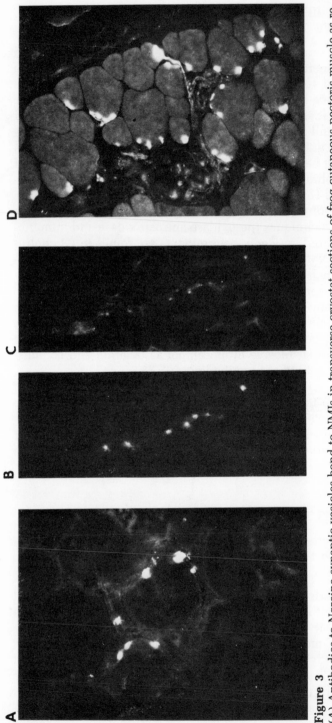

Figure 3

(A) Antibodies to Narcine synaptic vesicles bond to NMJs in transverse cryostat sections of frog cutaneous pectoris muscle as revealed here by fluorescein-conjugated goat anti–rabbit IgG. (B) Unstimulated (resting) frog cutaneous pectoris muscles bind little or no synaptic vesicle antibodies in the living state. After incubating the living muscle with antiserum, the preparation was quick-frozen and cryostat sections were then stained with a fluorescein-conjugated second antibody. (C) Rhodamine-conjugated, α-bungarotoxin-labeled endplates in the same transverse cryostat section as B, thus verifying positions of NMJs that did not bind synaptic vesicle antibody in whole mount. (D) Lanthanum-stimulated frog cutaneous pectoris muscles bind synaptic vesicle antibodies in the living state. Lanthanum-treated preparations were incubated with antiserum and then quick-frozen and sectioned. Transverse cryostat sections were then stained with a fluorescein-conjugated second antibody.

bungarotoxin. This toxin is thought to increase presynaptic membrane permeability.

3. When whole mounts of the cutaneous pectoris are treated in the living state with the trivalent cation lanthanum, which produces the complete release of all synaptic vesicles from the terminals, about 70% of the NMJs are labeled (Fig. 3D).

These results strongly suggest that a substance present on the inside of the synaptic vesicle is exposed to the antibodies only when synaptic vesicles are inserted into the plasma membrane of the presynaptic terminal during exocytosis. We predict, but have not yet proven, that the conserved antigens are determinants on the luminal face of the synaptic vesicle. These could be one or more of the six unique vesicle proteins or the putative proteoglycan.

Sepharose or polyacrylamide beads with goat anti−rabbit IgG serum attached can be bound to synaptic vesicles coated with anti−synaptic vesicle antiserum. They also bind to synaptosomes from electric organ that have been precoated with anti−synaptic vesicle antibodies (G.P. Miljanich et al., in prep) (Fig. 4). The binding can be monitored either by cytoplasmic choline acetyltransferase or by electron microscopy. The presynaptic membrane is then obtained by releasing the contents by osmotic lysis. This membrane is largely free of contamination by ACh receptors, $Na^+K^+ATPase$, and major membrane proteins of the electric organ. The plasma membrane is also quite different from the synaptic membrane, on the basis of two criteria. First, in two-dimensional gel analyses, the protein compositions show little similarity. Second, antisera raised to the isolated plasma membrane recognize antigens in the nerve terminal that are not on synaptic vesicles. These sera also cross-react with antigenic determinants at the frog neuromuscular junction. Unlike the antisera to synaptic vesicles, however, the antibodies to electric organ presynaptic plasma membrane bind to the outside of the resting nerve terminals (A. Brasier, unpubl.). No binding is detectable after denervation.

CONCLUSION

• Using a purified synaptic vesicle fraction from a marine ray to immunize rabbits, highly specific polyclonal antibodies to the vesicles are obtained. Although these antibodies are not of monoclonal origin, they are extremely valuable in quantifying the amount of antigen from various tissues, in following the fate of vesicle antigens, and in isolating the presynaptic plasma membrane. They have also been invaluable in setting up the screens for nerve-terminal-specific monoclonal antibodies now being characterized.

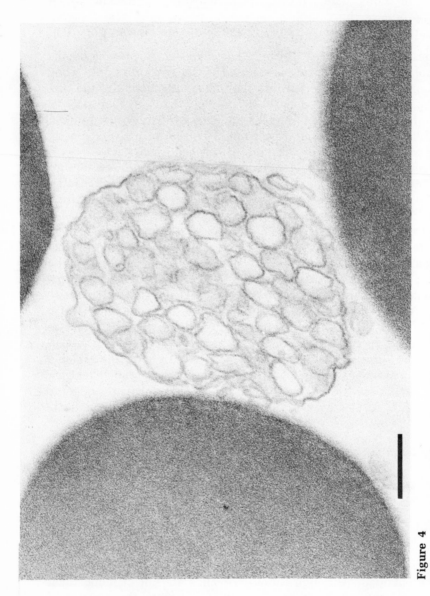

Figure 4

Electric organ synaptosome bound to antibody-coated beads. Synaptosomes were incubated first with rabbit anti–synaptic vesicle antiserum, then with goat anti–rabbit Ig–coated polyacrylamide beads ("Immunobeads," BioRad). The sample was fixed in glutaraldehyde and postfixed in OsO$_4$. Bar is 0.2 μm.

REFERENCES

Carlson, S.S., and R.B. Kelly. 1980. An antiserum specific for cholinergic synaptic vesicles from electric organ. *J. Cell Biol.* **87**:98.

Hooper, J.E., S.S. Carlson, and R.B. Kelly. 1980. Antibodies to synaptic vesicles purified from *Narcine* electric organ bind a subclass of mammalian nerve terminals. *J. Cell Biol.* **87**:104.

Sanes, J.R., S.S. Carlson, R.J. von Wedel, and R.B. Kelly. 1979. Antiserum specific for motor nerve terminals in skeletal muscle. *Nature* **280**:403.

von Wedel, R.J., S.S. Carlson, and R.B. Kelly. 1981. Transfer of synaptic vesicle antigens to the presynaptic plasma membrane during exocytosis. *Proc. Natl. Acad. Sci.* **78**:1014.

Wagner, J.A., and R.B. Kelly. 1979. Topological organization of proteins in an intracellular secretory organelle: The synaptic vesicle. *Proc. Natl. Acad. Sci.* **76**:4126.

Wagner, J.A., S.S. Carlson, and R.B. Kelly. 1978. Chemical and physical characterization of cholinergic synaptic vesicles. *Biochemistry* **17**:1199.

Monoclonal Antibodies to Synaptic Membranes and Vesicles

WILLIAM D. MATTHEW,* LOUIS F. REICHARDT,*† and LARISA TSAVALER†

Departments of *Biochemistry and †Physiology
University of California
San Francisco, California 94143

• One of the goals of our laboratory is to obtain more-detailed knowledge of the molecular composition of the synapse. We hope to understand the function of the different molecules found in the synapse and use this information to obtain a finer understanding of the molecular changes that occur during synaptogenesis. Ultimately, this knowledge should clarify the factors that enable the nervous system to be formed with such precision.

Biochemical studies on synapses, central or peripheral, have been severely limited by inadequate purification procedures for synaptic membranes, junctions, densities, or associated organelles. The preparations described in the literature are contaminated with non-synaptic and nonneuronal material. Most contain a very heterogeneous population of synapses from many different cell types. The only convincing studies on localization of molecules within a synapse have used immunocytochemical methods.

Immunological probes that recognize particular types of neurons, synapses, or other structures would provide purification procedures based on different principles than the physical methods currently available and therefore should enable synapses and neurons to be completely purified for more-definitive biochemical studies. They would also be useful for determining the functions of individual antigens and could be used as markers to dissect the different steps in synaptogenesis. Since different monoclonal antibodies recognize single antigenic determinants in a complex immunogen, hybridomas provide a method for neurobiologists to obtain highly specific antisera to components of the very impure biochemical preparations

163

currently available. Consequently, the problems encountered in using classical immunological procedures with heterogeneous immunogens are avoided. In this paper we demonstrate that monoclonal antibodies raised against brain synaptic junction and membrane preparations show great specificity for the different cell types and organelles in the nervous system; we also provide one example of the use of these antibodies in purifying an organelle crucial for normal synaptic function.

PREPARATION OF SYNAPTIC JUNCTIONS AND ANTIBODIES

• We have made monoclonal antibodies to synaptic membrane and synaptic junction preparations in the hope that some of these antibodies will be specific for synapses. These preparations were purified by standard biochemical methods. Adult rat brain was homogenized and hypotonically lysed; then a synaptic-membrane-enriched fraction was isolated on a sucrose gradient. As illustrated in Figure 1 (left), these membranes consist of resealed presynaptic membrane, a piece of postsynaptic membrane, synaptic densities, and cleft material. When these membranes are extracted in Triton X-100, 90% of the protein is solubilized, leaving an intact junctional complex (Fig. 1, right). In the population of antibodies directed against these preparations, we anticipate finding neuronal surface markers, synaptic markers, and antibodies to contaminating membranes from other cell types.

To prepare the hybridoma, cell lines, BALB/c mice were given

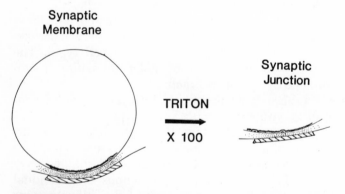

Figure 1
Rat brain fractions used to immunize mice. Synaptic membranes were prepared by the procedure of Jones and Matus (1974). Junctional complexes were prepared from synaptic membranes by the procedure of Wang and Mahler (1976).

two separate injections. After the spleen cells were fused to the NS1 nonsecreting myeloma cell line, the cells were plated at a clonal dilution in selective medium. We used a standard solid-phase radioimmunoassay to screen the antibodies produced in culture. Clones that bound synaptic membrane were screened against kidney, liver, spleen, and thymus membranes. Only the clones whose antibodies appeared to be brain-specific were maintained. Single cells from each cell line have been used to establish permanent cell lines. We have worked with 80 such cell lines whose antibodies selectively recognize brain. In this selection, we have found antibodies that recognize different cell types and organelles.

ANTISERA THAT DISTINGUISH CELL TYPES IN THE NERVOUS SYSTEM

• In Figure 2 are examples of monoclonal antibodies that distinguish the major cell types of the central and peripheral nervous systems (CNS and PNS, respectively). Figure 2A shows an unfixed dorsal root ganglion (DRG) culture stained with antiserum 22. The fluorescent probe demonstrated that this antibody recognized a proteoglycan on the surface of a sensory neuron. The antibody did not bind the fibroblasts and Schwann cells that surround this neuron and are visible in phase-contrast optics. Figure 2B is a photograph of an oligodendrocyte whose surface was stained by serum 9. The cell was counterstained by anti-galactocerebroside antiserum to verify that it was an oligodendrocyte. No other living cell types in cultures from the CNS or PNS were stained by this antiserum. Figure 2C is a fluorescent photomicrograph showing the binding of antiserum 17 to the intermediate filaments in an astrocyte. Our monoclonal collection thus distinguishes the major cell types in the nervous system. Our results also indicate that different neuronal types have antigenic differences, since many of our sera recognize neuronal subpopulations (data not shown). Intriguingly, many of the neuronal surface antigenic determinants appear to be on glycosaminoglycans.

ANTIBODIES THAT BIND SYNAPSES AND SYNAPTIC VESICLES

• A number of antibodies show very localized binding to synaptic regions of brain. Some of the antigens are exposed on the cell surface, whereas others are internal antigens. In the following discussion, we concentrate on two of these antisera as examples of how monoclonal sera are characterized and applied to studies in the nervous system.

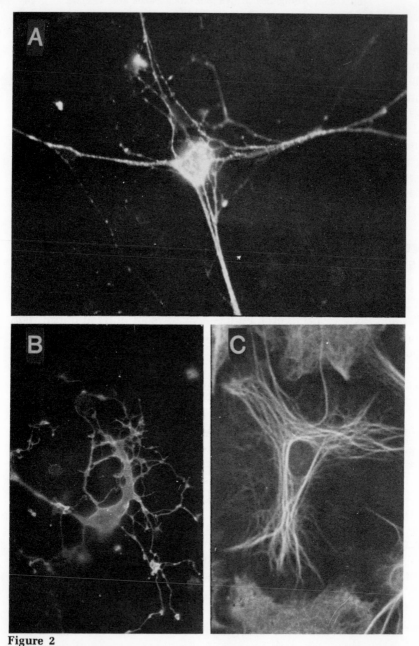

Figure 2
Indirect immunofluorescence showing the binding of monoclonal antibodies to primary dissociated cells in culture. (*A*) A newborn DRG culture; antibody 22 binds a proteoglycan on the surface of the neuron in this culture. (*B* and *C*) Newborn cerebral cortex cultures. In *B* antibody 9 binds to the surface of an oligodendrocyte. In *C* the cells were permeabilized before antibody incubation. This photograph shows that antibody 17 binds to intermediate filaments in an astrocyte.

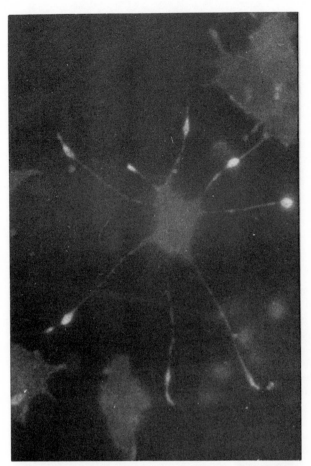

Figure 3
Indirect immunofluorescence on PC12 cells grown
with nerve growth factor. After the cells have been
permeabilized, antibodies 30 and 48 bind to varicosities and growth cones.

Identification of the Antigens

Two different antibodies, 30 and 48, stain the varicosities and growth
cones of PC12 cells that have been made in response to nerve growth
factor (NGF). To see binding (Fig. 3), the cells must be permeabilized.
These two antibodies are of different allotypes and arose from separate clones (data not shown); however, they recognize the same
protein. Part of the evidence for this conclusion is presented in
Figure 4, autoradiographs of a Burridge gel (Burridge 1978). In this
experiment, rat brain was solubilized in SDS-mercaptoethanol. After
the proteins were separated by gel electrophoresis, they were fixed in

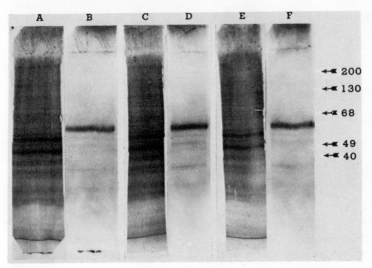

Figure 4
Identification of antigens. Synaptic plasma membranes were dissolved in SDS-mercaptoethanol and fractionated in 10% polyacrylamide gels. The antigens were identified by initial incubation with the monoclonal antibody and subsequent incubation with ^{125}I-labeled goat anti–mouse immunoglobulins (Burridge 1978). (A, C, and E) Coomassie-blue-stained gel lanes; also shown are the autoradiographs of gels treated with (B) serum 30, (D) serum 48, and (F) both serum 30 and serum 48.

methanol-acetic acid. Once the gel was neutralized in Tris buffer, it was incubated in monoclonal antibody, washed, put into ^{125}I-labeled goat anti–mouse IgG, washed, dried, and autoradiographed. The results show that serum 30 (Fig. 4B), serum 48 (Fig. 4D), and sera 30 and 48 together (Fig. 4F) bind a single protein band at m.w. 65,000. This is a minor protein band that is not visible in the Coomassie-blue-stained slabs used for autoradiography (Fig. 4A,C,E). These two antisera also compete with each other for binding in radioimmunoassays (data not presented). Serum 30 can completely block the binding of serum 48, and vice versa. Since these antibodies bind the same molecular-weight protein and block the binding of each other, they must be against the same protein.

Localization of the Antigens to Synaptic Vesicles

To see whether this protein is associated with synapses, we used immunohistochemical techniques to localize the antigen in sections of the rat cerebellum. The cerebellum is very convenient because it is a layered structure with defined cells and types of synapses that can be recognized in the microscope. Figure 5 is a photomicrograph of a fixed, frozen section of rat cerebellum that has been incubated with serum 30. Goat anti–mouse IgG serum was used to cross-link the bound mouse antibodies to rat peroxidase-antiperoxidase (PAP) complexes. Following the procedures of Sternberger (1979), we added 3,3'-diaminobenzidine (3,3',4,4'-tetraaminobiphenyl) (DAB) as a substrate for the peroxidase, and a brown, insoluble reaction product can be visualized in both the light and electron microscopes. This section has not been counterstained, so only the DAB reaction product appears dark. The molecular layer, which contains many small synapses, is heavily stained with tiny punctate spots. The Purkinje cell bodies show no product. In the granule cell layer are comparatively large, dark depositions of reaction product corresponding to the large glomerular synaptic complexes found in that region of the cerebellum. In sections counterstained with toluidine blue (not shown), the peroxidase reaction product is found in large intercellular spaces between granule cells. In both the molecular layer and granule cell layer, the pattern of reaction product deposition suggests that this antigen is localized to the vicinity of synapses.

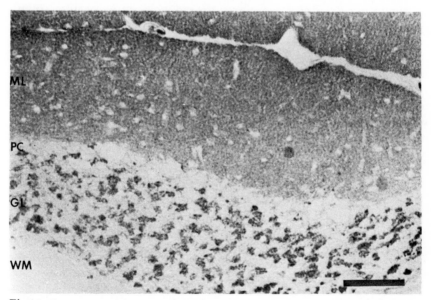

Figure 5
Immunocytochemical localization of the antigen. Light microscopy of a representative cerebellar section that was tested for serum-30 immunoreactivity is shown (bar, 100 μm). This section was not counterstained. The peroxidase reaction product appears dark. Abbreviations indicate major cerebellar layers: ML (molecular layer); PC (Purkinje cell layer); GL (granule cell layer); and WM (white matter).

To localize the protein bound by these two antisera more defini-
tively, we needed the resolution of the electron microscope. For these
experiments, the antibody binding and PAP reaction were completed
using 50-μm vibratome sections. Then ultrathin sections were made
from embedded material. To be certain the thin sections were maxi-
mally penetrated by the antisera, they were cut parallel and close to
the surface of the thick sections. Figure 6A is a photomicrograph of a
section through two glomeruli in the granule cell layer. The large,
dark terminals are mossy fiber endings. The surrounding smaller
endings are the terminals of Golgi neurons. A granule cell soma and
nucleus are shown in the same photograph. In each case, the DAB
reaction product is associated with synaptic vesicles. Figure 6B
shows a similar section through the molecular layer. Every one of the
small terminals found in this region of the cerebellum is filled with
reaction product. A more highly magnified photograph of one terminal (Fig. 6C) shows that the DAB reaction product is on the outer
surface of the vesicles.

Immunoprecipitation of Synaptic Vesicles and Their Internal Contents

To obtain more-definitive evidence for the localization of this protein,
we immunoprecipitated the organelles containing the antigen from a
crude, hypotonically lysed brain homogenate and identified those
organelles in the electron microscope. A section of this lysed homogenate is shown in Figure 7A. This section contains a very heterogeneous mixture of membrane profiles, including partially lysed synaptosomes, mitochondria, and free synaptic vesicles. After incubation
with antibody for 60 minutes, membranes were separated from unbound antibody by centrifugation. In the final step the organelles
containing bound antibody were precipitated with protein A coupled
to 2–10-μm polyacrylamide beads. The beads were fixed, embedded,
sectioned, and examined in the electron microscope. Figure 7B is a
representative photograph of the profiles precipitated by normal

Figure 6
High-resolution localization of serum-30 immunoreactivity in the cerebellum.
These electron micrographs show sections of the granule cell layer in A (bar,
2 μm) and molecular layer in B (bar, 2 μm), with a higher-magnification
micrograph of a parallel fiber terminal in C (bar, 0.5 μm). The peroxidase
reaction product appears dark. In the granule cell layer (A), both the large
mossy fiber terminals (MF) and surrounding Golgi type-II terminals (GT)
have depositions of reaction product; (N) granule cell nucleus. In the molecular layer (B), every terminal contains reaction product. Deposition of reaction
product around vesicles is apparent in C.

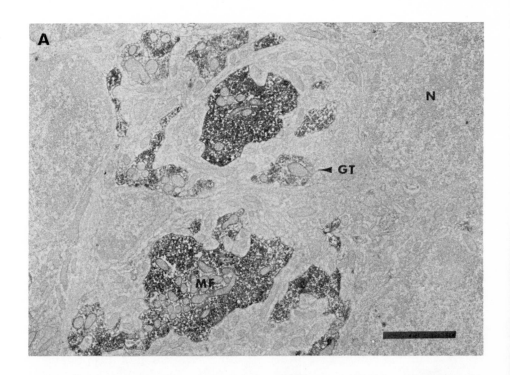

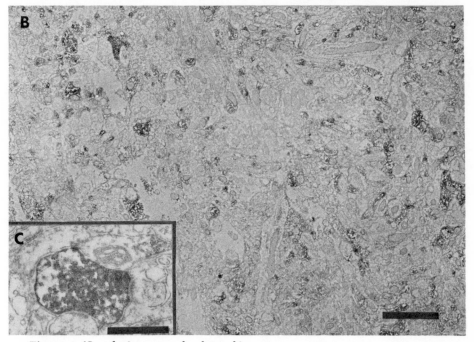

Figure 6 (*See facing page for legend.*).

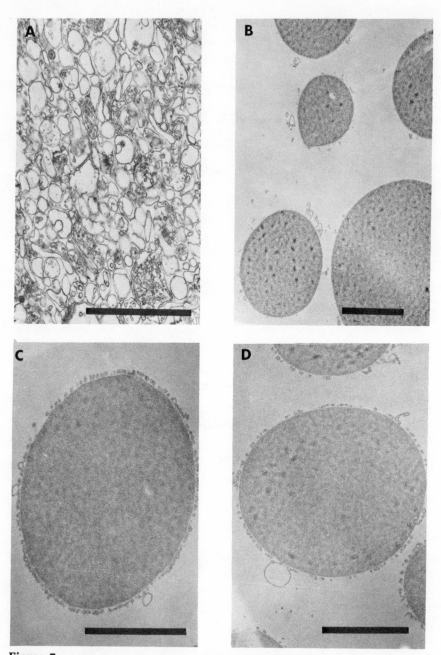

Figure 7
Membrane profiles immunoprecipitated on protein A–acrylamide beads. The experimental procedure has been described by Ito and Palade (1978). (A) An electron micrograph of a sectioned crude brain homogenate; (B) an electron micrograph of a sectioned acrylamide bead with attached membrane profiles immunoprecipitated with normal mouse serum; (C and D) profiles precipitated with serum 30 (bars, 1 μm).

mouse serum. Only an occasional piece of membrane is found on the surface of the polyacrylamide beads. In experiments with monoclonal sera not directed against membrane antigens, we have found even fewer profiles on these beads (data not shown). In contrast, when serum 30 is used (Fig. 7C,D), a large number of uniformly sized vesicle profiles, the size of brain synaptic vesicles, are found on the outside surface of the beads. Plasmalemma profiles are rare, and mitochondrial profiles are absent. Clearly, this single immunoprecipitation step is capable of significantly purifying vesicles from a crude homogenate. We have compared the ratio of vesicle profiles to other profiles in the homogenate and immunoprecipitated material. This procedure gives us a 30-fold enrichment in vesicle profiles.

To demonstrate that intact vesicles can be precipitated with their internal contents, we incubated PC12 cells in [³H]norepinephrine (NE) prior to homogenization. Patterson et al. (1976) have shown that vesicular, but not cytoplasmic, [³H]NE is retained on Millipore filters, presumably because vesicle proteins bind to nitrocellulose. Using this assay to estimate the [³H]NE remaining in vesicles after homogenization, we found that 95% of the vesicular [³H]NE could be immunoprecipitated on acrylamide beads (Table 1a). In Table 1b are the results of a similar experiment in which the cells were grown for 5 days in [¹⁴C]leucine and for 1 hour in [³H]NE. In a homogenate, the [³H]NE to acid-precipitable [¹⁴C]leucine ratio was defined as 1:1. After immunoprecipitating the vesicles with serum 30, this ratio was increased to 10:1. In Table 1a, we show that 50% of the [³H]NE was released from vesicles during the 4-hour incubation period in our immunoprecipitation protocol, so vesicle membrane components were probably purified 20-fold. Since PC12 cells contain large numbers of vesicles, a 20-fold purified preparation may be close to homogeneity, but this has not yet been proved.

Distribution of the Protein in Secretory Tissues

From Figure 6 it is evident that this antigen is present in all or virtually all the vesicles in the cerebellum, which includes many types of excitatory (e.g., mossy fiber) and inhibitory (e.g., Golgi terminal) synapses. Thus, it seemed likely the antigen was distributed very widely in the nervous system. To quantitate the amount of antigen in different homogenates, we used an adsorption assay in which the amount of tissue required to remove half of a limiting dilution (1 ng) of antibody was measured with a series of dilutions of the homogenate. After removing membranes and adsorbed antibody molecules, the remaining antibody was titered in a solid-phase radioimmunoassay. In Table 2, the relative amounts of antigen in a variety of nonsecretory, secretory, and neurosecretory tissues are normalized to the amount found in a whole rat brain homogenate. Two

Table 1

Immunoprecipitation of [³H]Norepinephrine from PC12 Homogenates

a. Efficiency of Immunoprecipitation of [³H]NE[1]

	Total cpm sampled	cpm bound to Millipore filter	cpm precipitated on beads
Cell homogenate (time 0)	5200	2100	–
Cell homogenate (4 hr, 20°C)	5200	940	–
Cell homogenate + antibody 30 (4 hr, 20°C)	5200	980	930

b. Immunoprecipitation of [³H]NE from a PC12 Homogenate Containing [¹⁴C]Leucine-labeled proteins[2]

	[³H]NE:[¹⁴C]leucine
Cell homogenate	1.0
Protein A–polyacrylamide bead	10.6

[1]10⁶ PC12 cells were incubated with 1 μCi [³H]NE for 80 min at 37°C (Patterson et al. 1976). Cells were homogenized in 1 ml of growth medium with a glass-Teflon homogenizer; then large debris was removed by centrifugation at 10,000g for 5 min. Aliquots were used to estimate the vesicular [³H]NE content by Millipore filtration (Patterson et al. 1976). Preparations were incubated at room temperature and samples removed and adsorbed to Millipore filters to determine the rate at which transmitter leaks out of these vesicles. Values are cited for 4 hr, the time required to complete the immunoprecipitation on beads. Aliquots were used for immunoprecipitations: 300-μl aliquots were mixed with 40 μg of each antibody, incubated for 100 min at 2°C, and adsorbed to immobilized protein A.

[2]PC12 cells were grown in the presence of [¹⁴C]leucine for 5 days prior to a 60-min incubation in [³H]NE. The ratio of [³H]NE to [¹⁴C]leucine was normalized to the value found in the homogenate, which has been defined as 1.0.

nonsecretory paradigms, extrajunctional diaphragm muscle and adrenal cortex, have little or no antigen (< 0.4% of the level in rat brain). All regions of the CNS examined — cerebral cortex, cerebellum, and superior colliculus — have comparable high levels of the antigen. Two neural-crest-derived tissues, the sympathetic ganglion and adrenal medulla, also have high levels of the antigen, and the antigen is also found in PC12, a neuronlike tumor derived from the neural crest.

In contrast, a variety of nonneuronal secretory tissues, such as salivary gland, have much lower levels of antigen, which may indicate that the protein either is present in low amounts on the secretory vesicles in these tissues or is restricted to a subpopulation of vesicles (e.g., those in the innervating nerve terminals). The antigen is found

Table 2
Quantitative Measurement of Antigen in Different Tissues

	% RSA[1]
Tissue homogenized	
Extrajunctional diaphragm muscle (rabbit)	<0.3
Adrenal cortex (bovine)	<0.4
Pancreas (rabbit)	0.9
Liver (rabbit)	0.9
Salivary gland (rabbit)	5.4
Anterior pituitary (bovine)	11.0
Superior cervical ganglion (rabbit)	27.0
Adrenal medulla (bovine)	76.0
Posterior pituitary (bovine)	86.0
Cerebral cortex (rabbit)	75.0
Cerebellum (rabbit)	60.0
Superior colliculus (rabbit)	50.0
Whole brain (rat)	100.0
Cell type homogenized	
Blood cells (rabbit)	<0.2
HIT (hamster pancreatic islet)	<0.5
AtT20 (mouse anterior pituitary)	5.0
GH3 (rat anterior pituitary)	12.0
PC12 (rat adrenal phaeochromocytoma)	26.0
PC12 grown in NGF	38.0

Aliquots of 76 ng/ml of ascites fluid 48 in 5% newborn calf serum in PBS (a dilution chosen to be limiting in the assay) were incubated with different concentrations of homogenized tissues for 12 hr at 4°C. The membranes were pelleted at 200,000g for 40 min in an airfuge. The residual antibody in the supernatant was measured in the solid-phase radioimmunoassay (Klinman 1972). The amount of tissue protein needed to adsorb 50% of the binding was recorded from inhibition curves. The inverse values were normalized to rat brain, which has been defined as 100% relative specific activity (RSA).

[1]RSA (relative specific activity) = antigen units per mg tissue/ antigen units per mg rat brain × 100.

in both posterior and anterior pituitary, even though the latter is not derived from neural tube or crest. The antigen is also found in two peptide-secreting cell lines, AtT20 and GH3, which are derived from the anterior pituitary, lending further evidence that the antigen is in anterior pituitary cells.

To summarize this and other data, the antigen has been found in every neuronal or neurosecretory tissue that we have examined, central or peripheral. By immune competition assay, it is almost certainly in every part of the nervous system. It is in the major terminals of the cerebellum (Fig. 6), which include both excitatory and inhibitory synapses. Similar immunohistochemical procedures have indicated that the antigen is also present in every synaptic layer of the hippocampus and spinal cord (data not presented). The antigen is present in putative glutaminergic and GABAnergic (γ-aminobutyric acid) terminals (cerebellar parallel fibers and Golgi type-II endings), catecholaminergic tissue (adrenal, PC12), serotonergic tissue (pineal), and cholinergic endings (presynaptic terminals in frog sympathetic ganglion, PC12). It is also found in a variety of peptidergic cells or terminals (the luteinizing-hormone-releasing hormone [LHRH] terminals in the frog sympathetic ganglion, growth-hormone-secreting GH3 cells, adrenocorticotropic hormone [ACTH]- and endorphin-releasing AtT20 cells, posterior and anterior pituitary). Although this is not proven, we believe that the 65,000-dalton protein is probably present on every neurosecretory vesicle.

Insertion of the Antigen at Sites of Exocytosis

In Figure 8 are light (A) and electron (B) microscope photographs that show the location of DAB reaction product in the rabbit adrenal medulla after incubation with serum 30. In Figure 8A it is evident that the reaction product is found in the adrenal medulla but not in the cortex. In Figure 8B the reaction product is found on the outer surface of chromaffin granules and on the inner surface of that portion of the plasmalemma that faces a sinusoidal space. In many micrographs, we have consistently seen reaction product on this surface but not on other portions of the plasmalemma, even though they are also closely apposed to chromaffin granules (see Fig. 8B). Therefore, we believe the reaction product marks sites of vesicle fusion. In this case, vesicles may have been trapped in the plasmalemma during the fixation procedure since others have also seen this phenomenon (Heuser 1978).

Quite possibly, the nonvesicular membrane profiles seen after immunoprecipitation with acrylamide beads (Fig. 7C,D) are inverted plasmalemma fragments containing the vesicle antigen since these profiles were always empty in contrast to the mitochondria and partially lysed synaptosomes that were prevalent in the initial homogenate (Fig. 6A). Fusion and trapping may occur during fixation or homogenization and may be the major reason for contamination of our vesicular preparations. Fortunately, plasmalemma fragments are predominantly larger than vesicles, and the two can be separated on controlled-pore glass columns. In preliminary experiments, it appears that combining a molecular sieving step with immunoprecipitation is a rapid and efficient way to purify synaptic vesicles.

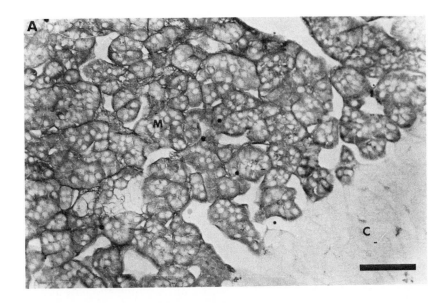

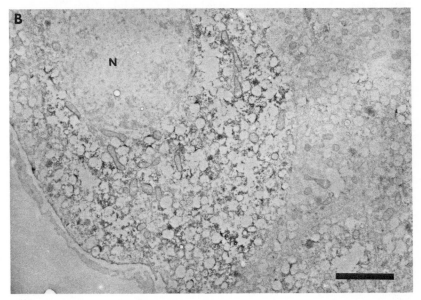

Figure 8

Localization of immunoreactivity in the adrenal medulla. Representative photomicrographs show the localization of serum-30 immunoreactivity in the adrenal gland. (A) A low-power photomicrograph that includes portions of both the adrenal cortex (C) and medulla (M); the peroxidase reaction is clearly found only in the medulla, where it is localized inside adrenal chromaffin cells (bar, 100 μm). (B) An electron micrograph of chromaffin cells; a thin deposition of reaction product outlines the chromaffin granules and the inside surface of sinusoidal portions of the plasmalemma (bar, 2 μm).

Table 3

Quantitative Measurement of Antigen in Different Vertebrate Species

Brain Homogenized	% RSA
Drosophila	<0.9
Chicken	77.0
Frog	86.0
Rabbit	87.0
Mouse	89.0
Rat	100.0
Cow	120.0
Shark	200.0

The procedure was as described in the notes to Table 2.

Evolutionary Conservation of the 65,000-dalton Protein

Table 3 shows the results of an experiment in which the amounts of antigen in different species were compared using the immune competition assay. Although antigen was not detected in fruit flies, high levels were found in shark, chicken, frog, and every mammal examined. Clearly, the antigen has persisted through several hundred million years of evolutionary divergence.

In fact, the 65,000-dalton protein has retained its molecular weight and the features of its conformation in these different species. The Burridge gel in Figure 9 shows that the antibody binds the same molecular-weight protein in each species. This particular autoradiograph has been overexposed to show antibody binding to two minor bands at 40,000 and 50,000 daltons. Although there are many possible explanations for these minor bands, it seems very likely that they are proteolytic fragments of the 65,000-dalton protein. If so, the protease-sensitive sites have also been preserved in the different species, suggesting that the major structural features of the protein are highly conserved.

SUMMARY

• We have isolated a series of monoclonal antibodies that distinguish the major cell types of the nervous system and recognize molecules concentrated at synapses. Concentrating on one example, we have identified a vesicle-specific protein that is probably on every neurosecretory vesicle and is clearly very highly conserved in vertebrate evolution. Since it is exposed on the outer surfaces of secretory granules, it could have a role in vesicle biogenesis, transport, exocytosis, recycling, or any other function common to both metabolite- and peptide-containing vesicles. We are initiating immunological and

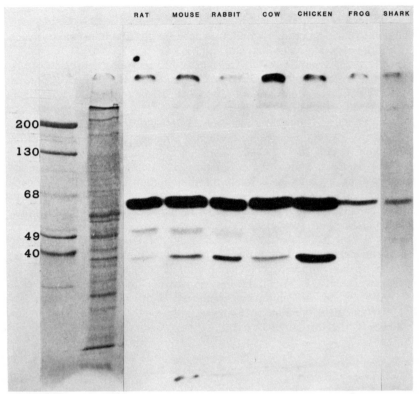

Figure 9
Identification of antigen in different vertebrate species. A whole brain was
dissolved in SDS-mercaptoethanol and processed as described in the legend to Fig. 4. Gel lanes containing protein standards and rat brain, both
stained with Coomassie blue, are shown at the left. The molecular weights
(in kilodaltons) of the protein standards are indicated. The different species used as sources for the brain homogenates are identified at the top of
appropriate lanes.

genetic experiments to determine its function. The antisera should be
very useful for purifying and characterizing vesicles and their contents as well as for monitoring development of nerve terminals during synaptogenesis.

ACKNOWLEDGMENTS

• Research was supported by grants to L.F.R. from the National
Science Foundation, Muscular Dystrophy Association, McKnight
Foundation, March of Dimes Birth Defects Foundation, and Wills
Foundation. L.F.R. is a Sloan Foundation Fellow.

REFERENCES

Burridge, K. 1978. Direct identification of specific glycoproteins and antigens in SDS gels. *Methods Enzymol.* **50:**54.

Heuser, J.E. 1978. Synaptic vesicle exocytosis and recycling during transmitter discharge from the neuromuscular junction. In *Transport of macromolecules in cellular systems* (ed. S.C. Silverstein), p. 445. Dahlem Konferenzen, Berlin.

Ito, A. and G. Palade. 1978. Presence of NADPH-cytochrome P-450 reductase in rat liver Golgi membranes. Evidence obtained by immunoabsorption method. *J. Cell Biol.* **79:**590.

Jones, D.H. and A.I. Matus. 1974. Isolation of synaptic plasma membranes from brain by combined flotation-sedimentation density gradient centrifugation. *Biochim. Biophys. Acta* **356:**276.

Klinman, N.R. 1972. The mechanism of antigenic stimulation of primary and secondary clonal precursor cells. *J. Exp. Med.* **136:**241.

Patterson, P.H., L.F. Reichardt, and L.L.Y. Chun. 1976. Biochemical studies on the development of primary sympathetic neurons in cell culture. *Cold Spring Harbor Symp. Quant. Biol.* **40:**389.

Sternberger, L.A. 1979. The unlabeled antibody peroxidase-antiperoxidase (PAP) method. In *Immunocytochemistry*, p. 104. Wiley, New York.

Wang, Y.-J. and H.R. Mahler. 1976. Topography of the synaptosomal membrane. *J. Cell Biol.* **71:**639.

Monoclonal Antibodies to Synaptosomal Membrane Molecules

ANGEL L. DE BLAS, NEIL A. BUSIS, and MARSHALL NIRENBERG

Laboratory of Biochemical Genetics
National Heart, Lung, and Blood Institute
National Institutes of Health
Bethesda, Maryland 20205

• Our objective has been to obtain monoclonal antibodies to molecules in synaptosome membranes that affect the formation or function of synapses.

GENERATION AND IDENTIFICATION OF HYBRIDOMAS

• Hybridoma cell lines synthesizing antibodies to a synaptosome plasma membrane (SPM) fraction (Jones and Matus 1974; De Blas and Mahler 1978) from 33-day-old rat cerebral cortices were obtained by fusion of P3-X63/Ag-8 mouse myeloma cells (Köhler and Milstein 1975) with spleen cells from BALB/c mice immunized with SPM as described by Galfre et al. (1977). A summary of fusion conditions and yields of hybridomas from two fusion experiments is shown in Table 1. Of the 428 hybridoma cell lines obtained, 50 cell lines were found that synthesize antibodies to SPM.

Hybridoma antibodies to SPM molecules were detected by an indirect radioimmunoassay based on the binding of affinity-purified rabbit $[^{125}I]F(ab')_2$ anti–mouse IgG to complexes of mouse hybridoma antibody and SPM antigen as described in the legend to Figure 1. The relations between the concentrations of antigen protein, hybridoma antibody, or rabbit $[^{125}I]F(ab')_2$ antibody fragment and total, nonspecific, and specific $[^{125}I]F(ab')_2$ bound are shown in Figure 1 A, B, and C, respectively.

Antibodies in ascites fluid harvested from hybridoma ascites tumors were used in the experiments shown in Figure 1; however, in other experiments antibodies secreted into the culture medium

Table 1

Generation of Hybridomas Synthesizing Antibodies to Rat Cerebral Cortex
Synaptosome Plasma Membranes

	Fusion	
Description	4	2
1. Immunize mice with 1.5 mg SPM protein IP[1] and 0.4 mg SPM protein IV[2] on day	0,8,24,37	0,8,14
2. Fusion on day	40	17
P3-X63/Ag-8 cells	20×10^6	40×10^6
immunized mouse spleen cells	100×10^6	100×10^6
feeder layer spleen cells	7.5×10^6	7.5×10^6
3. $\dfrac{\text{Antibodies to synaptosomes}}{\text{Total hybridoma cell lines}}$	$\dfrac{35}{296} = 12\%$	$\dfrac{15}{132} = 11\%$
4. $\dfrac{\text{Wells with hybridomas}}{\text{Total wells innoculated}}$	$\dfrac{296}{660} = 45\%$	$\dfrac{132}{708} = 19\%$

[1]IP = Intraperitoneal injection.
[2]IV = Intravenous injection in tail vein.

by hybridoma cells sometimes were employed. The amount of $[^{125}\text{I}]\text{F(ab'})_2$ that bound specifically to the [hybridoma antibody • rat cerebral cortex antigen] P2 fraction was proportional to the amount of protein in the range of 0 to 700 μg (Fig. 1A). Specifically bound $[^{125}\text{I}]\text{F(ab'})_2$ also was proportional to 4-6F5 hybridoma antibody concentration in the range of 0 to 1 μl of ascites fluid (Fig. 1B). Under the conditions used, half-maximal and maximal specific $[^{125}\text{I}]\text{F(ab'})_2$ binding values were obtained in the presence of 0.9 and 3 μM $[^{125}\text{I}]\text{F(ab'})_2$, respectively (Fig. 1C). Usually when antibodies in ascites fluid were used, conditions were adjusted so that specific $[^{125}\text{I}]\text{F(ab'})_2$ binding was approximately 67% of the maximum specific binding; reaction mixtures contained limiting concentrations of antigen, excess hybridoma antibody, and 1.28 μM $[^{125}\text{I}]\text{F(ab'})_2$.

EFFECTS OF HYBRIDOMA ANTIBODIES ON SYNAPSES

• The effects of hybridoma antibodies on clonal neuroblastoma $\times$ glioma NG108-15 hybrid cells synapsing with rat myotubes were studied by measuring the frequency of spontaneous miniature end-plate potentials (MEPPs) of myotubes by means of intracellular microelectrodes (Nelson et al. 1976) (Table 2). Each MEPP presumably represents the myotube response to acetylcholine secreted from a single NG108-15 vesicle. Four to six antibodies were pooled and tested together. In the presence of antibodies in set 1 or 2, the number

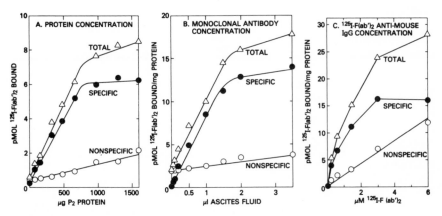

Figure 1
The effects of antigen protein concentration (A), hybridoma antibody concentration (B) and concentration of rabbit [^{125}I]F(ab')$_2$ (C) directed against mouse IgG on total, nonspecific, and specific [^{125}I]F(ab')$_2$ binding to rat cerebral cortex P2 particulate protein. (△) Total [^{125}I]F(ab')$_2$ bound in the presence of hybridoma antibody 4-6F5; (o) nonspecific binding in the presence of antibody (light chains) synthesized by parental P3-X63/Ag-8 cells; (●) specific [^{125}I]F(ab')$_2$ binding; that is, total [^{125}I]F(ab')$_2$ bound in the presence of hybridoma antibody, minus nonspecific [^{125}I]F(ab')$_2$ bound in the presence of antibody synthesized by P3-X63/Ag-8 cells, and minus [^{125}I]F(ab')$_2$ bound to plastic in the absence of antigen protein. Each stage-1 reaction mixture contained the following components, except where specified, in a final volume of 100 μl: 160 μg (B) or 320 μg (C) rat cerebral cortex synaptosomal-mitochondrial P2 particulate protein (De Blas and Mahler 1978); 2 μl 4-6F5 hybridoma antibody in ascites fluid or 2 μl P3-X63/Ag-8 antibody; 100 μg gelatin; and 98 μl Dulbecco's phosphate-buffered saline (PBS) (pH 7.4). Reaction mixtures in 96-well polyvinylchloride plates previously incubated with 1 mg gelatin per ml PBS were incubated for 45 min at 3°C, pellets were recovered by centrifugation (3,500g for 5 min at 3°C), washed 3 times (175 μl PBS per wash), and recovered each time by centrifugation. Each stage-2 reaction mixture contained the following components, except where specified, in a final volume of 50 μl: washed [hybridoma antibody • particulate antigen] complex; 1.28 μM rabbit [^{125}I]F(ab')$_2$ (approximately 75,000 cpm per well) directed against mouse IgG (heavy and light chains); 500 μg bovine serum albumin; 50 μg gelatin; and 50 μl PBS (pH 7.4). Reaction mixtures were incubated for 45 min at 3°C, antibody•antigen complexes were washed and recovered by centrifugation 3 times, as described above, and bound radioactivity was determined.

of MEPPs per minute increased 2.7- and 1.9-fold, respectively; myotube hyperpolarization also was found. However, myotube hyperpolarization also was observed in the presence of antibodies in set 7 with no effect on the frequency of MEPPs. Smaller increases in MEPP frequency were found with antibody sets 3, 4 (myotube depolariza-

Table 2

Effects of Pooled Antibodies on Synapses between NG108-15 Hybrid Cells and Rat Myotubes

Pooled antibodies	Mean MEPPs per min per myotube	Mean myotube resting membrane potential (mV)	% myotubes with synapses	No. of myotubes tested
P3-X63/Ag-8	14 ± 2	−59 ± 1	77	30
None	12 ± 2	−58 ± 1	68	38
Set 1	38 ± 6‡	−67 ± 2†	95	20
Set 2	27 ± 8*	−64 ± 1	90	10
Set 3	23 ± 4	−62 ± 2	100	10
Set 4	21 ± 5	−52 ± 1†	75	20
Set 5	19 ± 3	−60 ± 1	90	10
Set 6	16 ± 4	−61 ± 2	90	10
Set 7	12 ± 3	−69 ± 3†	80	10
Set 8	9 ± 2	−62 ± 3	90	10
Set 9	9 ± 3	−56 ± 1	80	10

Synapses between NG108-15 hybrid cells and rat striated myotubes were detected by recording miniature endplate potentials (MEPPs) from myotubes by means of intracellular microelectrodes (Nelson et al. 1976). Myoblasts from the hind limbs of newborn Fisher rats were dissociated and cultured for 7–8 days in 35-mm petri dishes (Nelson et al. 1976). The monolayers of well-differentiated, multinucleated myotubes obtained were approximately 20% confluent and were relatively free of other cell types. NG108-15 cells (2×10^5) were then added to each dish with myotubes, and the cells were cocultured for 4 days in 1.5 ml of medium A (88% Dulbecco's modification of Eagle's minimal medium, 10% horse serum incubated for 20 min at 56°C to inactivate complement, 0.1 mM hypoxanthine, and 0.016 mM thymidine) supplemented with 10 μM prostaglandin E_1, 1 mM theophylline, and with 4 or 6 hybridoma antibodies in ascites fluid that had been incubated for 20 min at 56°C to inactivate complement. Each hybridoma antibody was diluted 800-fold (final concentration); P3-X63/Ag-8 ascites fluid was diluted 200- or 122-fold when used as the control for 4 or 6 pooled hybridoma antibodies, respectively. Antibodies and media were replaced daily.

Myotubes with 3 or more MEPPs per min were considered innervated. Only recordings from muscle cells with stable resting membrane potentials more negative than −45 mV, without artifacts, were used. Two hr before testing myotubes for synapses, the medium was changed to medium A without serum, adjusted to 3.8 mM $CaCl_2$ and 129 μM choline chloride, and supplemented with 10 μM prostaglandin E_1, 1 mM theophylline, 5 μM tetrodotoxin (to prevent spontaneous myotube action potentials), and the appropriate antibodies at twice the concentrations stated above. Antibodies were pooled as follows: (Set 1) 2-2G7, 2-4D7, 2-4H3, 2-5C7, 2-7B8, and 2-8B11; (Set 2) 4-7E2, 4-7G9, 23E10, and 24D6; (Set 3) 4-5G4, 4-1C10, 4-2A8, 4-2D2, 4-2H3, and 4-3B3; (Set 4) 4-4C3, 4-4G7, 4-5A4, 4-4A7, 4-5F1, and 4-5G11; (Set 5) 4-5H2, 4-6C12, 4-6F5, and 4-6H2; (Set 6) 4-5G9, 4-6C2, 4-6F9, and 4-7A2; (Set 7) 4-2A6, 4-5A3, 4-5C3, and 4-5C5; (Set 8) 2-1G8, 2-2C3, 2-7F11, and 2-4B4; and (Set 9) 2-8B5, 4-1A8, 4-1G1, and 4-3G6.

Mean values ± S.E. are shown in the second and third columns. P values for the differences between the mean values found with pooled hybridoma antibodies and the P3-X63/Ag-8 control values based on a two-tailed t-test are as follows: *$0.01 < P < 0.05$; †$0.001 < P < 0.01$; ‡$P < 0.001$.

tion also found), and 5, but not with other sets of antibodies tested. These results suggest that some of the antibodies affect the permeability of cells to ions and the rate of acetylcholine secretion from NG108-15 cells.

The rates of spontaneous and evoked acetylcholine secretion from the hybrid cells decrease in the absence of extracellular Ca^{++} ions (McGee et al. 1978; Nelson et al. 1978; De Blas et al. 1981; H. Higashida et al.; M. Wilson et al.; both in prep.). Therefore, each antibody in set 1 was tested separately for effects on MEPP frequency of myotubes and $^{45}Ca^{++}$ uptake by neuroblastoma × liver NBr10-A hybrid cells (Table 3). NBr10-A cells also form many synapses with muscle cells (H. Higashida et al., in prep.) and were used in $^{45}Ca^{++}$ uptake studies because fewer cells were lost when these cell monolayers were washed as compared with NG108-15 monolayers. At 5 mM K^+, $^{45}Ca^{++}$ uptake by NBr10-A cells was increased 56% by antibody 2-5C7 and 23% by antibody 2-4H3. Depolarization of NBr10-A cells by 80 mM K^+ resulted in activation of voltage-sensitive Ca^{++} channels and increased $^{45}Ca^{++}$ uptake by cells (Rotter et al. 1979); but the antibodies tested had no effect on depolarization-dependent uptake of $^{45}Ca^{++}$ ions. MEPP frequencies also were increased in the presence of hybridoma antibody 2-5C7 or 2-4H3; however, these antibodies did not affect myotube membrane potentials (not shown). The other four antibodies in set 1, when tested separately, did not affect $^{45}Ca^{++}$ uptake or myotube resting potentials (not shown). The demonstration that antibody 2-5C7 or 2-4H3 increased both $^{45}Ca^{++}$ uptake by hybrid cells and the frequency of MEPPs suggests that antibody-dependent enhancement of $^{45}Ca^{++}$ uptake by the hybrid cells increased their rate of acetylcholine secretion. The antigens recognized by antibodies 2-5C7 and 2-4H3 were detected in liver and kidney as well as in the central nervous system (see below). Specific binding sites for antibody 2-5C7, but not for antibody 2-4H3, were detected on NG108-15 cells (not shown).

In other experiments not shown here, rates of $^{45}Ca^{++}$ uptake at 5 and 80 mM K^+ were not affected by 27 hybridoma antibodies, each tested separately. Preliminary results suggest that 4 additional antibodies affect $^{45}Ca^{++}$ uptake, but further work is needed to confirm these observations.

ANTIBODY SPECIFICITY FOR RAT TISSUES

· The specificities of antibodies secreted by cultured hybridoma cells into the medium for antigens associated with crude membrane preparations from rat cerebral cortex, liver, and kidney are shown in Table 4. Of the 13 hybridoma antibodies tested, 4 bound to cerebral cortex

Table 3

Effect of Antibodies on $^{45}Ca^{++}$ Uptake by NBr10-A Cells and on the Frequency of Myotube Responses at Synapses

	pmoles $^{45}Ca^{++}$ uptake by NBr10-A cells per min per mg protein		Mean MEPPs per min per myotube
Antibody	5 mM K+	80 mM K+	
P3-X63/Ag-8	613	1704	18
2-5C7	956	1775	42
2-4H3	753	1706	44

The assay for $^{45}Ca^{++}$ uptake is described by Rotter et al. (1979). Briefly, NBr10-A hybrid cells were incubated for 5 days in medium A with 1 mM dibutyryl cAMP in multiwell dishes (2 cm² surface area per well) and then for 20 hr in fresh medium containing 0.8 mM L-[3,4-³H]valine (250 cpm per nmole) and for 2 hr in medium with unlabeled valine. Cells were equilibrated for 30 min at 37°C in solution B (114 mM NaCl; 5mM KCl; 50 mM HEPES, sodium salt [pH 7.4]; 1.8 mM CaCl; 0.8 mM MgCl; 0.9 mM NaH₂PO₄; 25 mM glucose; 0.1 mM hypoxanthine; 0.001 mM aminopterin; 0.016 mM thymidine; 1 mM dibutyryl cAMP; and the antibody specified diluted 100-fold [heat-inactivated ascites fluid]). Then the medium was replaced with 0.5 ml of solution B per well supplemented with $^{45}CaCl_2$ (usually 3500 cpm per nmole $^{45}CaCl_2$) and the antibody specified diluted 100-fold, or with solution B adjusted to 80 mM KCl and 39 mM NaCl and supplemented with $^{45}CaCl_2$ and antibody diluted 100-fold. Cells were incubated for 60 sec, washed 4 times (2 ml each wash) at 4°C with solution B without dibutyryl cAMP, hypoxanthine, aminopterin, thymidine, or antibody. Cells were solubilized in 0.7 ml of 1 N NaOH, an aliquot was neutralized, and $^{45}Ca^{++}$ and ³H radioactivities were determined and corrected for spillover. Portions of samples from 24 wells were pooled, the protein concentration was determined by a modification of the method of Lowry et al. (1951), and ³H and $^{45}Ca^{++}$ radioactivities were determined. The amount of protein per well was calculated from the mean cpm per mg of ³H-labeled protein found for the pooled samples (53,900 cpm per mg ³H-labeled protein) and the cpm of ³H-labeled protein found for the sample from each well. Each $^{45}Ca^{++}$ uptake value shown is the mean of 3 to 6 values obtained with replicate wells. Experimental procedures for determining the effects of antibodies on MEPP frequency are described in Table 2.

membranes but did not bind or bound only slightly to liver and kidney membranes; 4 antibodies bound both to cerebral cortex and liver membranes but not to kidney membranes; 1 antibody bound to cerebral cortex and kidney membranes but only slightly to liver membranes; and 4 antibodies bound to membranes from the 3 tissues tested. In most cases the amount of [¹²⁵I]F(ab′)₂ that bound specifically to cerebral cortex membranes was higher than that found with liver or kidney membranes. These results show that most of the antibodies tested exhibit tissue specificity.

Additional results on antibody specificity were obtained with antibodies in ascites fluid harvested from mice bearing hybridoma ascites tumors (Table 5). Six antibodies, 4-1A8, 4-7E2, 4-6C2, 2-7B8, 4-3G6, and 4-2A6, bound to a greater extent to cerebral cortex synaptosomal plasma membranes than to a cerebral cortex 9000g P2 parti-

Table 4

Specificity of Antibodies in Hybridoma Culture Medium for Rat Cerebral Cortex, Liver, and Kidney

| Experiment no. | Antibody | pmoles [^{125}I]F(ab')$_2$ bound specifically per mg protein | | |
		cerebral cortex	liver	kidney
1.	P3-X63/Ag-8	(1.0)	(1.0)	(1.0)
	4-1C11	3.7	0.1	0
	2-2C3	3.0	0.1	0
	4-6C2	0.4	0.1	0
	2-4B4	0.3	0	0
	4-5G9	4.2	0.6	0
	4-3G6	1.3	0.3	0
	2-7B8	0.8	0.2	0
	2-2G7	0.2	0.5	0
	4-5G11	0.4	0.1	0.2
	4-2A6	7.1	2.7	0.9
	2-4D7	5.5	2.3	1.1
2.	P3-X63/Ag-8	(3.0)	(3.0)	(1.5)
	2-4H3	22.6	21.2	14.2
	4-6F5	29.7	23.6	6.6

Each stage-1 reaction mixture contained antibody in 175 μl of conditioned medium that had been used for culture of hybridoma cells and 128 μg of 9000g particulate protein (P2 fraction [De Blas and Mahler 1978]) from rat cerebral cortex, liver, or kidney. Reaction mixtures were incubated for 45 min at 3°C and then washed as described in the legend to Fig. 1. In experiments 1 and 2, each stage-2 reaction mixture contained the components described in the legend to Fig. 1 and 640 or 1280 nM [^{125}I]F(ab')$_2$ (3829 or 1494 cpm per pmole [^{125}I]F(ab')$_2$), respectively. Reaction mixtures were incubated for 45 min at 3°C and then membranes were washed and recovered as described in the legend to Fig. 1. Each value is the mean of duplicate determinations. Specific [^{125}I]F(ab')$_2$ binding is shown; i.e., total [^{125}I]F(ab')$_2$ bound, minus [^{125}I]F(ab')$_2$ bound nonspecifically in the presence of medium conditioned by P3-X63/Ag-8 cells, minus [^{125}I]F(ab')$_2$ bound to plastic in the absence of antigen protein. Values for [^{125}I]F(ab')$_2$ bound nonspecifically in the presence of medium conditioned by P3-X63/Ag-8 cells are enclosed within parentheses and have been subtracted from other values shown.

culate fraction. Antibodies 4-5A3 and 4-1A8 exhibit regional specificity within the nervous system, since the antibodies bound to antigens in cerebral cortex and cerebellum, but little or no specific binding of antibody to retina was detected. No specific binding of these antibodies to liver membranes was detected. Also, little or no specific binding of antibodies 4-1A8, 4-5C3, and 2-8B11 to kidney membranes was detected.

Table 5

Specificity of Antibodies in Ascites Fluid for Rat Tissues

| Antibody | Cerebral cortex[1] | | Cerebellum[1] | Retina[1] | Liver[1] | Kidney[1] |
	synaptosome plasma membranes	9000g pellet				
P3-X63/Ag-8	(2.9)	(2.8)	(4.9)	(2.2)	(2.8)	(2.5)
4-5A3	5.9	6.5	9.6*	0‡	0‡	1.2‡
4-1A8	4.3†	1.6	2.5*	0.2‡	0‡	0‡
4-5C3	2.6†	5.0	5.3	2.2†	1.5†	0.1‡
2-8B11	2.1	2.1	–	–	0.4*	0
4-7E2	1.9†	0.8	0.5	0.6	0.3†	1.0
4-6C2	6.5‡	1.7	0.5*	0.5†	–	–
2-7B8	8.6†	6.3	6.7	6.1	–	–
4-3G6	4.6†	3.3	3.1	2.3	–	–
4-2A6	5.2*	4.0	3.1*	2.8†	1.6†	1.0†
2-8B5	6.8	6.8	4.6*	1.3‡	1.3‡	3.4
2-4D7	8.5	8.6	12.5†	7.8	4.0†	2.6‡
2-5C7	3.7	4.9	6.5†	2.4‡	9.5†	15.1‡
4-4C3	8.9	9.7	–	–	8.8	5.4
2-2C3	–	9.8	8.1	4.1†	–	–

Reaction mixture components are described in the legend to Fig. 1. Nonspecific [^{125}I]F(ab′)$_2$ binding values in the presence of P3-X63/Ag-8 ascites fluid, shown enclosed within parentheses, have been subtracted from the other values shown; [^{125}I]F(ab′)$_2$ bound to plastic in the absence of antigen protein also was subtracted from the values shown. Rat cerebral cortex synaptosomal plasma membranes were prepared as described previously (Jones and Matus 1974; De Blas and Mahler 1978); other fractions tested were 9000g P2 pellet fractions (De Blas and Mahler 1978). Each value shown is the mean of 5–8 experiments with duplicate or triplicate determinations in each experiment. P values are given when specific [^{125}I]F(ab′)$_2$ binding values found with the cerebral cortex 9000g pellet fraction differed significantly from values obtained with other fractions based on a paired two-tailed t-test within each experiment. * $0.01 < P < 0.05$; † $0.001 < P < 0.01$; ‡ $P < 0.001$.

[1]Units: pmoles [^{125}I]F(ab′)$_2$ bound specifically per mg protein.

As shown in Table 6, five antibodies were found that bound to a greater extent to a cerebral cortex membrane fraction from young adult rats than to the corresponding fraction from 17-day embryos. Other antibodies tested bound equally to embryo and adult cerebral cortex membranes (not shown).

Most, but not all, of the antibodies that bound to synaptosomal membranes also bound specifically to NG108-15 neuroblastoma × glioma hybrid cells. Treatment of NG108-15 cells with dibutyryl cAMP for 5 days shifts the cells to a more "differentiated" state and increases the number of synapses with myotubes (Nelson et al. 1976, 1978; H. Higashida et al., in prep.), cell membrane excitability (H.

Table 6

Antibody Binding to Rat Embryo and Adult Cerebral Cortex Membranes as a Function of Developmental Age

| Antibody | pmoles [^{125}I]F(ab')$_2$ bound specifically per mg protein | |
	17-day embryo	33-day adult
P3-X63/Ag-8	[1.2] ± 0.1 (4)	[2.8] ± 0.1 (8)
2-8B11	0.1 ± 0.1 (2)	2.1 ± 0.3 (3)
4-5C3	1.3 ± 0.2 (8)	5.0 ± 0.4 (5)
4-1A8	0.5 ± 0.1 (3)	1.6 ± 0.1 (8)
4-5A3	2.2 ± 0.2 (2)	6.5 ± 0.3 (8)
2-2C3	3.2 ± 0.3 (4)	9.8 ± 0.5 (4)

Nonspecific [^{125}I]F(ab')$_2$ binding values in the presence of P3-X63/Ag-8 antibody (ascites fluid) are enclosed within brackets; these values have been subtracted from the other values shown. Nonspecific [^{125}I]F(ab')$_2$ binding to plastic in the absence of antigen also was subtracted. Mean values are shown ± S.E.; the number of experiments is given in parentheses. Duplicate or triplicate assays were performed in each experiment. Seventeen-day rat embryo or 33-day adult rat cerebral cortex 9000g P2 pellet fractions were assayed as described in the legend to Fig. 1.

Higashida et al., in prep.), voltage-sensitive Ca^{++} channel activity (Rotter et al. 1978), and spontaneous and depolarization-dependent rates of acetylcholine secretion (McGee et al. 1978; Nelson et al. 1978; De Blas et al. 1981; H. Higashida et al.; M. Wilson et al.; both in prep.). Treatment of NG108-15 cells with 1 mM dibutyryl cAMP for 5 days increased 1.5- to 2.0-fold the specific binding of antibodies 4-6F5 and 4-2A6 to NG108-15 membranes but did not affect the specific binding of other antibodies tested (not shown).

In collaborative studies, F. Hirata and J. Axelrod have shown that one of the hybridoma antibodies, 4-4C3, is directed against lipomodulin (Hirata et al. 1981), a protein inhibitor of phospholipase A2 (Hirata et al. 1980).

CONCLUSIONS

• Fifty hybridoma cell lines were obtained that synthesize antibodies to molecules in rat cerebral cortex synaptosomal membrane preparations. Some of the antibodies bind to antigens in synaptosome membrane preparations that were not detected in liver or kidney. Two antibodies were found with regional specificity within the nervous system. These antibodies bind to molecules in cerebral cortex and cerebellar membrane fractions, but few or no antigenic sites were detected in retina fractions. Antigenic differences between embryonic and adult cerebral cortex membranes also were detected with certain antibodies. In addition, antibodies were found that affect synaptic transmission presynaptically by increasing $^{45}Ca^{++}$ uptake and acetylcholine secretion at synapses, monitored indirectly by determining MEPP responses of myotubes. Postsynaptic effects of antibodies were also found that result in myotube hyperpolarization or depolarization.

ACKNOWLEDGMENTS

• We thank Maria Shih and Linda Anderson for expert assistance in $^{45}Ca^{++}$ uptake experiments and Marty Green and Beth Todd for skillful preparation of the manuscript.

REFERENCES

De Blas, A. and H.R. Mahler. 1978. Studies on nicotinic acetylcholine receptors in mammalian brain. Characterization of a microsomal subfraction enriched in receptor function for different neurotransmitters. *J. Neurochem.* **30**:563.

De Blas, A., M. Adler, P. Chiang, G. Cantoni, M. Shih, and M. Nirenberg. 1981. Novel inhibitors of phosphatidylcholine synthesis, calcium action potential channels, and synapses. *Proc. Natl. Acad. Sci.* (in press).

Galfre, G., S.C. Howe, C. Milstein, G.W. Butcher, and J.C. Howard. 1977. Antibodies to major histocompatibility antigens produced by hybrid cell lines. *Nature* **266**:550.

Hirata, F., E. Schiffmann, K. Venkatasubramanian, D. Salomon, and J. Axelrod. 1980. A phospholipase A_2 inhibitory protein in rabbit neutrophils induced by glucocorticoids. *Proc. Natl. Acad. Sci.* **77**:2533.

Hirata, F., R. Del Carmine, C.A. Nelson, J. Axelrod, E. Schiffmann, A. Warabi, A.L. De Blas, M. Nirenberg, V. Manganiello, M. Vaughan, S. Kumagai, I. Green, J.L. Decker, and A.D. Steinberg. 1981. Presence of autoantibody for phospholipase inhibitory protein, lipomodulin, in patients with rheumatic diseases. *Proc. Natl. Acad. Sci.* **78**:3190.

Jones, D.H. and A.I. Matus. 1974. Isolation of synaptic plasma membrane from brain by combined flotation-sedimentation density gradient centrifugation. *Biochim. Biophys. Acta* **356**:276.

Köhler, G. and C. Milstein. 1975. Continuous cultures of fused cells secreting antibody of predefined specificity. *Nature* **256**:495.

Lowry, O.H., N.J. Rosebrough, A.L. Farr, and R.J. Randall. 1951. Protein measurement with the folin phenol reagent. *J. Biol. Chem.* **193**:265.

McGee, R., P. Simpson, C. Christian, M. Mata, P. Nelson, and M. Nirenberg. 1978. Regulation of acetylcholine release from neuroblastoma × glioma hybrid cells. *Proc. Natl. Acad. Sci.* **75**:1314.

Nelson, P., C. Christian, and M. Nirenberg. 1976. Synapse formation between clonal neuroblastoma × glioma hybrid cells and striated muscle cells. *Proc. Natl. Acad. Sci.* **73**:123.

Nelson, P.G., C.N. Christian, M.P. Daniels, M. Henkart, P. Bullock, D. Mullinax, and M. Nirenberg. 1978. Formation of synapses between cells of a neuroblastoma × glioma hybrid clone and mouse myotubes. *Brain Res.* **147**:245.

Rotter, A., R. Ray, and M. Nirenberg. 1979. Regulation of calcium uptake in neuroblastoma or hybrid cells—A possible mechanism for synapse plasticity. *Fed. Proc.* **38**:476.

Monoclonal Antibodies to the Nicotinic Acetylcholine Receptor

DARIA MOCHLY-ROSEN, MIRY C. SOUROUJON, ZELIG ESHHAR, and SARA FUCHS

Department of Chemical Immunology
The Weizmann Institute of Science
Rehovot, Israel

• Myasthenia gravis (MG) is an autoimmune disease of humans. Much about its likely pathogenesis has been learned from the animal model for the disease, experimental autoimmune myasthenia gravis (EAMG). In 1973, Patrick and Lindstrom observed that immunization of rabbits with the purified acetylcholine receptor (AChR) from the electric organ of the electric eel *Electrophorus electricus* resulted in a condition mimicking the electromyographic and clinical manifestations of MG. Since the rabbit sera contained antibodies to the eel AChR, they proposed that in EAMG, antibodies that cross-react with rabbit AChR bind to the receptors at the neuromuscular junction (NMJ) and interfere with synaptic transmission. To look further into this possibility, we have been using polyclonal sera and monoclonal antibodies raised against the intact and modified AChR to identify the immunological determinants responsible for the myasthenic activity of the AChR.

Before the advent of the methodology for producing monoclonal antibodies to a selected immunogen, we used polyclonal sera raised against the purified AChR of the electric ray *Torpedo californica* (Aharonov et al. 1977) and chemically modified or denatured AChR preparations (RCM-AChR) (Bartfeld and Fuchs 1977, 1978, 1979a). Recently, we have converted to the use of the more specific and potentially more informative monoclonal antibodies.

POLYCLONAL ANTIBODY STUDIES

Two Acetylcholine Receptor Modifications Are Antigenically Distinct

• The derivatives of the *T. californica* AChR used in this study and their agonist-binding properties and EAMG induction capabilities are summarized in Table 1. Not surprisingly, RCM-AChR shows antigenic characteristics that are different from those of native AChR. This is easily visualized in an immunodiffusion assay (Fig. 1) (Bartfeld and Fuchs 1977). Using rabbit polyclonal serum against AChR and another serum raised against RCM-AChR, the AChR and RCM-AChR bind in the same manner to anti-RCM-AChR serum, whereas there is only partial cross-reactivity between anti-AChR and RCM-AChR. This suggests the presence of an antibody in the anti-AChR serum against some determinants that do not exist on RCM-AChR. Apparently, determinants in the AChR molecule were abolished by the denaturation process. In particular, since RCM-AChR does not bind cholinergic ligands, the cholinergic-binding site appears to be severely altered by denaturation.

In addition to the loss of determinants on RCM-AChR, there are no determinants expressed on the intact AChR that become immunopotent after denaturation (Bartfeld and Fuchs 1979b). In Figure 2, the separation of the anti-AChR serum into two fractions is shown. This is done by passing the serum over an immunoabsorbant column (Sepharose covalently bound to RCM-AChR). The effluent and the eluate are collected. The binding specificities of these two fractions are determined by an inhibition assay, in which unlabeled antigens are used to inhibit the binding of ^{125}I-labeled AChR to: (A) the unfractionated anti-AChR serum, (B) the effluent from the column, or (C) the eluate of the column. RCM-AChR and AChR are used as inhibitors in this assay. From this polyclonal anti-AChR serum, a fraction that binds only to the intact AChR is obtained from the effluent (anti−native AChR antibodies). The antibodies in the eluate (anti−denatured AChR antibodies) that bind avidly to RCM-AChR also completely bind to AChR; no antibodies are present that bind only to RCM-AChR.

In another example of antigenic relationship, the interaction between the trypsinized receptor (T-AChR) and the two other AChRs

Table 1
Characterization of Two AChR Derivatives

Derivative	Modification	Binding of cholinergic ligands	Induction of EAMG
RCM-AChR	denaturation by reduction and alkylation in 6 M guanidine[1]	no	no
T-AChR	trypsinization[2]	yes	yes

[1]Bartfeld and Fuchs (1977, 1978).
[2]Bartfeld and Fuchs (1979a).

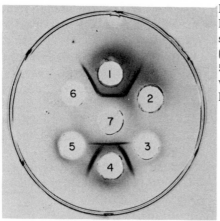

Figure 1
Immunodiffusion of anti-RCM-AChR serum (well 1) and anti-AChR serum (well 4) with RCM-AChR (wells 2, 3, 5) and AChR (wells 6, 7). (Reprinted, with permission, from Bartfeld and Fuchs 1977.)

was examined, using the anti–denatured AChR and the anti–native AChR sera obtained from the immunoabsorbant column. This was done by looking at the inhibition of ^{125}I-labeled AChR binding to either anti–native AChR (Fig. 3a) or anti–denatured AChR sera (Fig. 3b) by AChR, T-AChR, and RCM-AChR (Bartfeld and Fuchs 1979a; Fuchs et al. 1979). The anti–native AChR antibodies cross-reacted strongly with T-AChR, but T-AChR bound very weakly to the anti–denatured AChR antibody fraction.

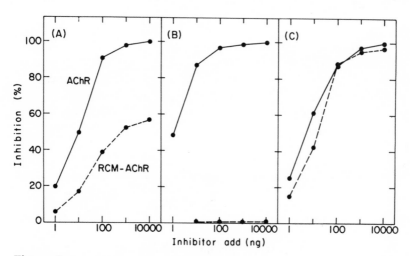

Figure 2
Inhibition of the binding of ^{125}I-labeled AChR to (A) unfractionated anti-AChR serum, (B) effluent serum, and (C) eluted antibody fraction by unlabeled AChR (————) and RCM-AChR (---------). (Reprinted, with permission from Bartfeld and Fuchs 1979b.)

In summary, the studies with polyclonal rabbit sera demonstrate two important results. First, all antibodies to RCM-AChR also bind to AChR; i.e., with the denaturation there are no new strongly immunogenic determinants formed on the receptor. In addition, RCM-AChR has no myasthenia-inducing capability; i.e., the myasthenic site(s) on the AChR seems to have been destroyed by the denaturation process. Second, anti–native AChR antibodies recognize sites on the T-AChR that apparently are not present on the RCM-AChR. Since T-AChR binds cholinergic ligands (see Table 1) and RCM-AChR does not, the cholinergic-binding site is thought to be preserved within this fragment of the AChR. Therefore, these preparations provide material for investigating the importance of the cholinergic-binding site in EAMG.

MONOCLONAL ANTIBODY STUDIES

Antibodies Bind Either to T-AChR or RCM-AChR but Not to Both

• Monoclonal antibodies with anti-AChR activity are prepared by hybridization of spleen cells from immunized mice and cells of the P3-NS1/1-Ag4-1 (NS1) nonsecreting plasmacytoma. Initially, C57BL/6

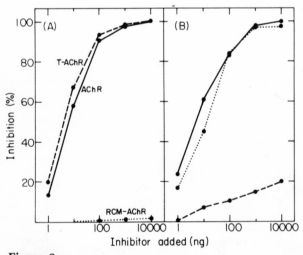

Figure 3
Antigenic specificity of T-AChR. Inhibition of the binding of ^{125}I-labeled AChR to anti-native-AChR antibodies (a) and to anti-denatured-AChR antibodies (b) by AChR (————), T-AChR (---------), and RCM-AChR (..........). (Reprinted, with permission, from Bartfeld and Fuchs 1979a.)

mice are injected twice with the purified *T. californica* AChR (Fuchs et al. 1976). To increase the number of specific antibody-forming cells, spleen cells from the immunized mice are transferred to lethally irradiated (800 rads) syngeneic mice. Following cell transfer, the recipient mice are injected intraperitoneally with purified AChR. The spleens of the recipient mice are removed four days later and afterwards fused with the nonsecreting plasmacytoma cells (Eshhar et al. 1979).

Those clones secreting antibodies binding to the purified AChR are selected by an indirect radioimmunoassay with radioiodinated AChR as the ligand and are developed to antibody-producing tumors following their injection into (BALB/c × C57BL/6)F1 mice. Using the ascites fluid as the antibody source, the specificities of the various antibody lines are assessed by radioimmunoassays (portrayed in Fig. 4 as both binding and inhibition curves). The AChR, RCM-AChR, and T-AChR are the radiolabeled ligands in these assays.

Some of the ascites fluid antibody titers against the AChR, RCM-AChR, or T-AChR are shown in Table 2. Some antibodies bind RCM-AChR, others bind T-AChR, and all bind strongly to the purified AChR. Interestingly, however, no antibody in this hybridization cross-reacts with both RCM-AChR and T-AChR. (This is in agreement with the previous data obtained using polyclonal sera raised against RCM-

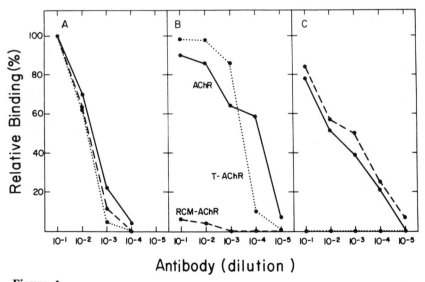

Figure 4
Antibody specificity of ascites fluids: binding experiments. Binding of ^{125}I-labeled AChR (————), RCM-AChR (---------), and T-AChR (..........) to (A) C57BL/6J anti-AChR serum; (B) 1.4; (C) 1.26. (Reprinted, with permission, from Mochly-Rosen et al. 1979.)

Table 2

Antibody Titers in Ascites Fluids (AF)

Sample	Antibody titer[1] toward		
	AChR	RCM-AChR	T-AChR
AF 1.3·	1.6×10^{-6}	0	4.0×10^{-8}
AF 1.4	1.0×10^{-5}	0	1.3×10^{-5}
AF 1.15	1.0×10^{-9}	0	1.0×10^{-8}
AF 1.20	1.4×10^{-7}	0	2.0×10^{-6}
AF 1.24	1.6×10^{-6}	0	2.0×10^{-6}
AF 1.26	2.0×10^{-7}	4.0×10^{-7}	0
AF 1.32	1.4×10^{-5}	0	1.8×10^{-5}
AF 1.34	1.6×10^{-6}	4.0×10^{-6}	0
AF 1.39	3.1×10^{-7}	8.0×10^{-7}	0
Immune serum (pool)	9.0×10^{-8}	5.3×10^{-8}	4.0×10^{-7}

Data from Mochly-Rosen et al. (1979).

[1] Antibody titers were determined by radioimmunoassay using goat anti-mouse Fab for precipitating the Ab-Ag complexes. Titers are expressed as moles of antigen precipitated per liter of serum.

AChR, which also do not exhibit cross-reactivity between the two modified receptors [see Fig. 3]). This effect is explicitly shown in Figure 4 for two representative monoclonal antibodies. The titrations of a C57BL/6J anti-AChR polyclonal serum (Fig. 4A) and two monoclonal antibodies (Fig. 4B,C) with either ^{125}I-labeled AChR, ^{125}I-labeled T-AChR, or ^{125}I-labeled RCM-AChR are indicated. Monoclonal antibodies 1.4 and 1.26 show a restricted specificity for either T-AChR or RCM-AChR, whereas the immune serum does not.

Monoclonal Antibody 5.5 Recognizes the Cholinergic-binding Site

We have produced one monoclonal antibody, 5.5, that does not bind to RCM-AChR. However, it does bind to T-AChR (which has a cholinergic-binding site and is capable of inducing EAMG in animals) and, even more important, it does not bind to AChR that has its cholinergic-binding site blocked by α-bungarotoxin (Table 3). Neither mouse anti-AChR serum nor the other anti-AChR monoclonal antibodies tested lacked binding to the α-bungarotoxin−AChR complex. Thus, specificity for the cholinergic-binding site seems to be present in monoclonal antibody 5.5.

Since monoclonal antibody 5.5 appeared to be directed against the α-bungarotoxin-binding site of AChR and since it bound specifically only to AChR preparations that retained their α-bungarotoxin-binding activity (AChR and T-AChR), we expected that it would also

Table 3
Specificity of Monoclonal Antibody 5.5

| | Antibody titer[1] toward | | | |
Antibody	AChR	T-AChR[2]	RCM-AChR[3]	α-bungaratoxin-AChR
5.5	6.4×10^{-8}	4.9×10^{-9}	—	—
Mouse anti-AChR	1.9×10^{-7}	1.9×10^{-7}	4.1×10^{-7}	3.2×10^{-7}

[1]Titers are expressed as moles of antigen precipitated per liter of serum.
[2]Trypsinated AChR.
[3]Denatured AChR obtained following reduction and carboxymethylation in 6 M guanidine HCl.

interfere with the binding of α-bungarotoxin to AChR. Indeed, as shown in Figure 5, monoclonal antibody 5.5 completely inhibited the binding of α-bungarotoxin to AChR. This inhibition was at least as effective as the one obtained by mouse anti-AChR serum. However, none of the other monoclonal antibodies with anti-AChR activity had a significant inhibitory effect, nor did a mixture of ten such antibodies (data not shown).

One very advantageous feature of monoclonal antibodies over polyclonal sera is that, because of their homogeneity, one can perform quantitative experiments looking at the competition between the binding of these antibodies and cholinergic ligands. This cannot be done with the heterogeneous population of polyclonal antibodies, with its broad spectrum of specificities for any individual antigen.

The binding of monoclonal antibody 5.5 to AChR was inhibited not only by α-bungarotoxin but also with other cholinergic ligands. The relative affinities of the various cholinergic ligands for AChR can be obtained through inhibition experiments with antibody 5.5 (Fig. 6). The concentrations of the various ligands necessary to give 50% inhibition of antibody-5.5 binding to ^{125}I-labeled-AChR obtained from Figure 6 compare favorably with the concentrations of the same ligands needed to produce a 50% inhibition of α-bungarotoxin binding to AChR (Table 4). These data strongly support the idea that monoclonal antibody 5.5 is directed against the cholinergic-binding site on the AChR, or at least against a site very closely associated with it.

CONCLUSION

• We have produced both polyclonal and monoclonal antibodies that recognize different determinants on the AChR. Monoclonal antibody

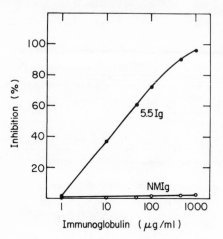

Figure 5
Inhibition of the binding of ^{125}I-labeled α-bungarotoxin to AChR by monoclonal antibody 5.5 (●) and by normal mouse immunoglobulins (○). ^{125}I-labeled α-bungarotoxin was incubated with the AChR for 30 sec at 4°C, following preincubation with the immunoglobulins.

5.5 binds directly to the cholinergic-binding site on the receptor, as shown by the fact that it competes strongly for cholinergic ligand binding. Because of their homogeneity, monoclonal antibodies are more useful than polyclonal antibodies in quantifying ligand-receptor interactions.

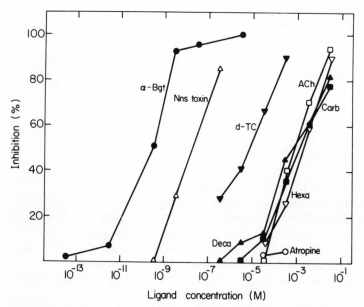

Figure 6
Inhibition of the binding of ^{125}I-labeled AChR to monoclonal antibody 5.5 by α-bungarotoxin (●), *Naja naja siamensis* α-neurotoxin (△), d-tubocurarine (▼), decamethonium (▲), carbamylcholine (■), hexamethonium (▽), acetylcholine (□), and atropine (○).

Table 4
Inhibition of the Binding of Anti-AChR Monoclonal Antibody 5.5 and of
α-Bungarotoxin to AChR by Cholinergic Ligands

Ligand	Inhibition of antibody-5.5 binding to AChR[1]	Inhibition of α-bungarotoxin binding to AChR[1]
α-Bungarotoxin	3×10^{-10}	1.5×10^{-10}
Naja naja siamensis toxin	1.3×10^{-8}	1×10^{-9}
d-Tubocurarine	6.2×10^{-6}	9×10^{-6}
Hexamethonium	1.6×10^{-3}	5.6×10^{-4}
Decamethonium	3.3×10^{-4}	5.0×10^{-5}
Carbamylcholine	0.5×10^{-4}	1.7×10^{-4}
Acetylcholine	6.1×10^{-4}	1.0×10^{-5}
Atropine	$> 10^{-2}$	1.2×10^{-2}

[1]Ligand concentration (M) at 50% inhibition.

In the future, we will continue to study the specificity of monoclonal antibody 5.5 by testing whether or not it binds to nicotinic
receptors in the central nervous system and whether the antibody can
recognize other macromolecules with a cholinergic-binding site. In
addition, we would like to look at the role of this antibody in EAMG
and hopefully determine whether the cholinergic-binding-site specificity of monoclonal antibody 5.5 is necessary or even sufficient by
itself to produce EAMG.

REFERENCES

Aharonov, A., R. Tarrab-Hazdai, I. Silman, and S. Fuchs. 1977. Immunochemical studies on acetylcholine receptor from *Torpedo californica*. Immunochemistry **14**:129.

Bartfeld, D. and S. Fuchs. 1977. Immunological characterization of an irreversibly denatured acetylcholine receptor. FEBS Lett. **77**:214.

————. 1978. Specific immunosuppression of experimental autoimmune
myasthenia gravis by denatured acetylcholine receptor. Proc. Natl.
Acad. Sci. **75**:4006.

————. 1979a. Active acetylcholine receptor fragment obtained by tryptic
digestion of acetylcholine receptor from *Torpedo californica*. Biochem. Biophys. Res. Commun. **89**:512.

————. 1979b. Fractionation of antibodies to acetylcholine receptor according to antigenic specificity. FEBS Lett. **105**:303.

Eshhar, Z., C. Blatt, Y. Bergman, and J. Haimovich. 1979. Induction of
secretion of IgM from cells of the B cell line 38C-13 by somatic cell
hybridization. J. Immunol. **122**:2430.

Fuchs, S., D. Nevo, R. Tarrab-Hazdai, and I. Yaar. 1976. Strain differences in
the autoimmune system of mice to acetylcholine receptors. Nature
263:329.

Fuchs, S., D. Bartfeld, Z. Eshhar, C. Feingold, D. Mochly-Rosen, D. Novick, M. Schwartz, and R. Tarrab-Hazdai. 1979. Immune regulation of experimental myasthenia. *J. Neurol. Neurosurg. Psychiatry* **43:**639.

Mochly-Rosen, D., S. Fuchs, and Z. Eshhar. 1979. Monoclonal antibodies against defined determinants of acetylcholine receptor. *FEBS Lett.* **106:**389.

Patrick, J. and J. Lindstrom. 1973. Autoimmune response to acetylcholine receptor. *Science* **180:**871.

Biochemical and Morphological Specificity of Retinal Amacrine Cells: Immunohistochemical Findings

HARVEY J. KARTEN and NICHOLAS BRECHA

Department of Psychiatry and Behavioral Sciences
Department of Neurobiology and Behavior
State University of New York
Stony Brook, New York 11794

• The general pattern of cellular organization of the vertebrate retina was clearly defined by the classic studies of Santiago Ramon Y Cajal (1893). Using the Golgi method, which selectively stains the entire cell, Cajal identified each of the major retinal cell types. These studies demonstrated the unique morphology of each of the major retinal classes of cells and revealed many detailed aspects of their interconnections. The major classes of retinal cells include distinctive photoreceptors, horizontal, bipolar, amacrine, and ganglion cells. In addition, the retina contains radially oriented glial (Müller) cells.

Within each retinal cell class, several distinct subcategories have been defined on the basis of differential morphological features, including the size and shape of their somata and the arborization pattern of their processes. For example, in the avian retina, at least five types of cones have been reported. These cells are distinguished on the basis of their content of different types of oil droplets in the outer segments as well as distinctive connections with appropriately matched bipolar cells. The morphology of cones and bipolar cells, however, is relatively homogeneous. In notable contrast, as shown in Figure 1, the amacrine and ganglion cell populations each consist of multiple morphological types.

Amacrine cells are unusual, as pointed out by Cajal, in that they appear to be typical neurons with varying, rich dendritic arborizations but without an axonal process. Cajal classified both amacrine and ganglion cells on the basis of their dendritic patterns of arborization as well as on the somewhat less satisfying distinction based on size of the somata (i.e., small, medium, and large). Both amacrine and ganglion cells arborize in the cell-free zone between them, the inner

203

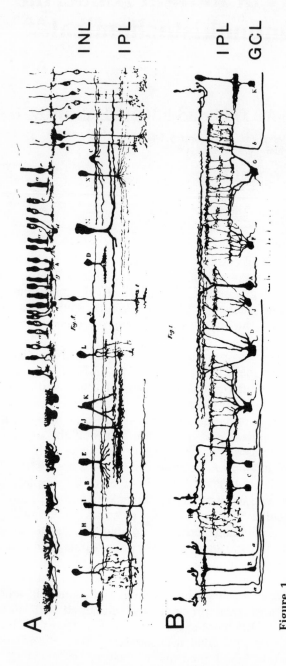

INL
IPL

IPL
GCL

Figure 1
Schematic drawing of Golgi-stained section of avian retina as summarized by Cajal. (A) Photoreceptors at the upper margin with horizontal cells, bipolar cells, and amacrine cells below them; (B) the pattern of ganglion cell arborizations in the IPL. (INL) Inner nuclear layer; (IPL) inner plexiform layer; (GCL) ganglion cell layer.

plexiform layer (IPL). Cajal subdivided the IPL into five nominal sublayers. Processes of both the amacrine and the ganglion cells were found to arborize in one sublayer (monostratified), two (bistratified), or several (multistratified) sublayers throughout the IPL. A variety of permutations of this pattern was noted, e.g., monostratified cells were located in layer 1, 2, 3, 4, or 5 of the IPL. Similarly bistratified cells were found to occur in any combination of layers of the IPL.

Recent research using histochemical and immunohistochemical methods has substantiated the morphological diversity of amacrine cells as observed with the Golgi method. These studies have concentrated on the localization of transmitters and "modulators" within the retina.

Using both monoclonal and conventional antibodies, we have studied the retinas of birds and other vertebrates, paying particular attention to the distribution of neuropeptides. Our work has mainly centered on the bird retina because of its extraordinary degree of differentiation and specialization. Figure 2 summarizes the results of

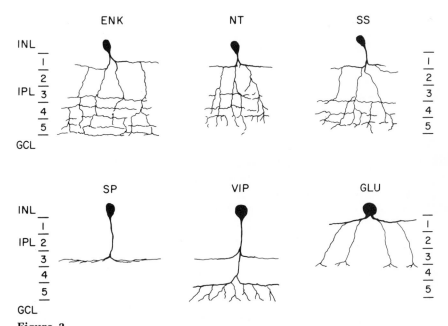

Figure 2
Schematic representation of peptidergic amacrine cells in the red field of the pigeon retina. The IPL contains five separate sublayers, as first described by Cajal. (INL) Inner nuclear layer; (IPL) inner plexiform layer; (GCL) ganglion cell layer; (ENK) enkephalinlike immunoreactive amacrine cells; (NT) neurotensinlike immunoreactivity; (SS) somatostatinlike immunoreactivity; (SP) substance P−like immunoreactivity; (VIP) vasoactive intestinal polypeptide-like immunoreactivity; (GLU) glucagonlike immunoreactivity.

our research of the past two years, demonstrating the patterns of immunohistochemical staining of the retina for various neuropeptides. To date we have confirmed the presence of six different peptides in the pigeon retina, including substance P (SP), enkephalin (ENK), vasoactive intestinal polypeptide (VIP), glucagon (GLU), neurotensin (NT), and somatostatin (SS). In all instances we should cautiously refer to the observed pattern of staining as being "peptide-like" staining in order to avoid the ambiguity consequent to the possible presence of other substances showing a common reactivity with the material of interest.

The most striking single observation of these studies is that only a single type of retinal neuron, the amacrine cell, stains for these peptides. The clarity of these findings is less clear-cut in many other classes of vertebrates; i.e., peptidelike staining is present in neurons located in the ganglion cell layer in several other classes of vertebrates. In general, the cells in the ganglion cell layer appear to be displaced amacrine cells, although further studies are needed to resolve their cell classification.

The second major feature of note is the morphological specificity of each type of peptidergic amacrine cell. As demonstrated in the schematic summary in Figure 2, each type of peptidergic amacrine cell possesses a unique morphology that in itself distinguishes it from other types of amacrine cells. In most instances this distinction is dramatically evident merely on the basis of the unique pattern of arborizations within the IPL. In the case of NT- and SS-containing cells, differences were observed in the arborization patterns in the proximal IPL: i.e., the processes of the SS-containing cells are more dense in lamina 4 than in lamina 3, whereas the processes of the NT-containing cells are equally dense in laminae 3 and 4.

A third indication of the distinctiveness of each population was observed when comparing the intercell spacing and density of each type of peptidergic amacrine cell. ENK-containing amacrine cells had an average spacing of 30 μm, whereas those of VIP were 64 μm, within the red-field zone of the retina. ENK, SS, NT, VIP, and GLU all showed their highest densities in the red field, whereas SP was lowest in density in the red field but highest in the yellow field of the inferior retina.

A fourth line of evidence of the distinctiveness of each type of peptidergic amacrine cell emerged from the use of the double-staining method. This was of particular value in attempting to compare the SS- and NT-containing cells, both of which stain amacrine cells with processes in layers 1, 3, and 4. Three adjacent sections were stained with anti-SS, anti-NT, and both anti-SS and anti-NT. The cells stained in each section were counted. The number of cells stained when both antisera were used together equaled the sum of the number stained with either antibody alone. Recently, more direct evidence has come from double staining of a single section with rabbit anti-NT and sheep anti-SS. These two antibodies can be distinguished by fluorescein- and rhodamine-labeled second layer immunoglobulins. This experiment demonstrated directly that NT and SS were found in two separate populations of cells.

The ability of specific antibodies against peptides to reveal and confirm the existence of distinct subsets of neurons within a seemingly uniform class of neurons is very exciting. Although the precise function of each of these peptides is unknown, these data provide a useful pointer to highlight and confirm differences otherwise evident only on the basis of random Golgi staining or serial electron microscope reconstructions. The further use of monoclonal antibodies will almost surely provide us with ever more refined probes to distinguish the differential morphologies of otherwise seemingly similar cells. Of perhaps even greater value, they provide a powerful tool for the biochemical identification of distinctive cell markers in the baffling complexity of the brain.

REFERENCES

Brecha, N., H.J. Karten, and C. Laverack. 1979. Enkephalin-containing amacrine cells in the avian retina: Immunohistochemical localization. *Proc. Natl. Acad. Sci.* **76:**3010.

Brecha, N., H.J. Karten, and C. Schenker. 1981. Neurotensin-like and somatostatin-like immunoreactivity within amacrine cells of the retina. *Neuroscience* (in press).

Cajal, S.R. 1893. La Retine des vertebres. *La Cellule* **9:**17.

Karten, H.J. and N. Brecha. 1980. Localization of substance P immunoreactivity in amacrine cells of the retina. *Nature* **283:**87.

Monoclonal Antibody F12A2B5: Reaction with a Plasma Membrane Antigen of Vertebrate Neurons and Peptide-secreting Endocrine Cells

GEORGE S. EISENBARTH, KAZUO SHIMIZU, MICHAEL CONN, ROBERT MITTLER, and SAMUEL WELLS

Duke University Medical Center
Durham, North Carolina 27710

• Experiments were previously undertaken to study cell-surface differentiation antigens of embryonic chick retina neurons, using monoclonal antibodies specifically reactive with neuronal plasma membranes (Eisenbarth et al. 1979). In view of the functional similarities between neurons and peptidergic endocrine cells (Gazdar et al. 1980), which include amine production, uptake, and decarboxylation mechanisms in addition to electrophysiologic properties such as activation of calcium channels for excitation-secretion coupling, the distribution of the neuronal antigen F12A2B5 was studied with a variety of endocrine tissues, tumors, and clonal cell lines.

PRODUCTION AND CHARACTERIZATION OF ANTIBODY F12A2B5

• Female BALB/c mice were immunized intraperitoneally on days 0 and 7 with 1×10^7 8-day embryonic chick retina cells fixed with 0.1% glutaraldehyde, in complete Freund's adjuvant, followed on day 37 by intravenous and intraperitoneal injections of 5×10^6 cells without adjuvant. On day 41, spleens were removed from two immunized mice, and 2×10^8 mechanically dissociated spleen cells were fused with 2×10^7 P3-X63/Ag-8 mouse myeloma cells in the presence of 0.8 ml of 50% polyethylene glycol 1000 (Baker), according to the method of Galfre et al. (1977). Hybridoma anti-retina antibodies were detected using either a complement-dependent cytotoxicity (^{51}Cr-release) assay or an ^{125}I-labeled staphylococcal protein-A radioassay (Schneider and Eisenbarth 1979). Tissue specificity of hybridoma

209

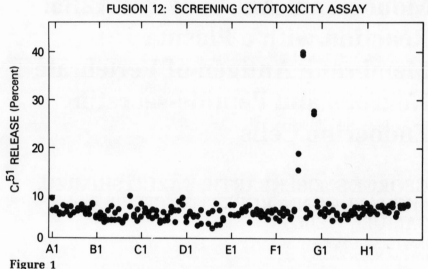

Figure 1

Complement-dependent microcytotoxicity assay (^{51}Cr-release) for anti-retina cell-surface antibodies produced by lymphocyte hybridomas.

antibody binding was established by quantitative adsorption and testing for residual anti-retina antibody activity, by indirect immuno-fluorescence microscopy, or by fluorescence-activated cell sorting. To facilitate distribution of cells, F12A2B5 clone 105 has been donated to the American Type Tissue Collection, Bethesda, Maryland.

Hybrid cell colonies were present two weeks after fusion in all 92 wells plated (2.2×10^6 cells per ml of medium per 2 cm^2 surface area). Of 92 tissue-culture supernatants, 42 contained antibody reactive with retina cells as detected by ^{125}I-labeled protein A, and 3 supernatants contained anti-retina antibody that was cytotoxic (Fig. 1). The hybridoma cell line F12A2B5 produced a cytotoxic antibody adsorbed by 8- or 16-day embryonic chick retina and brain, but not by liver, skeletal muscle, heart, kidney, or erythrocytes (Fig. 2). The antigen was also detected in human and bovine brain and the periph-eral nervous system (chick dorsal root ganglion).

ANTIBODY A2B5 LABELS CELL BODIES BUT NOT PROCESSES IN RETINA

• By indirect immunofluorescence, antibody A2B5 labeled cryostat sections of chick neural retina, with distinctive localization to the cell soma in the photoreceptor cell layer, inner nuclear layer, and gangli-on cell layer without labeling the outer or inner plexiform (synaptic) layers (Fig. 3). Similar binding to cell bodies but not processes was observed with short-term monolayer cultures of dissociated retina cells (Fig. 4). The antigen was detected on the soma of phase-bright, process-forming cells but not on flat, epithelioid cells that may represent Müller cells in culture. Antigen A2B5 was identified, however, on both the soma and processes of cultured chick dorsal root ganglion cells. Thus, localization to the cell soma is not an invariant property of the antigen.

ANTIGEN A2B5 IS A TETRASIALOGANGLIOSIDE

• Characterization of antigen A2B5 employed the inhibition of A2B5-dependent cytotoxicity. The antigen was sedimented by centrifugation at 100,000g for 30 minutes and was found to be resistant to heat and trypsin but sensitive to neuraminidase. The antigen was soluble in chloroform/methanol (2:1) and partitioned into the methanol/water phase of a Folch preparation, exhibiting the solubility properties of a ganglioside. Competition experiments were therefore performed with a variety of gangliosides (Fig. 5). A tetrasialoganglioside (GQ) fraction from bovine brain (Ledeen and Yu 1978), provided by P. Fishman

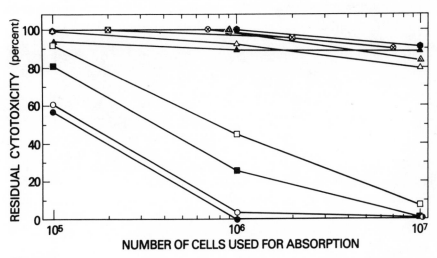

Figure 2
Residual cytotoxicity of antibody A2B5 following absorption with different numbers of cells from embryonic chick tissues: (●) 8-day brain; (○) 16-day brain; (■) 8-day retina; (□) 16-day retina; (▲) 8-day liver; (△) 16-day liver; (▲) 16-day muscle; (⊛) 16-day heart; (⊠) 16-day kidney; (●) 16-day erythrocytes.

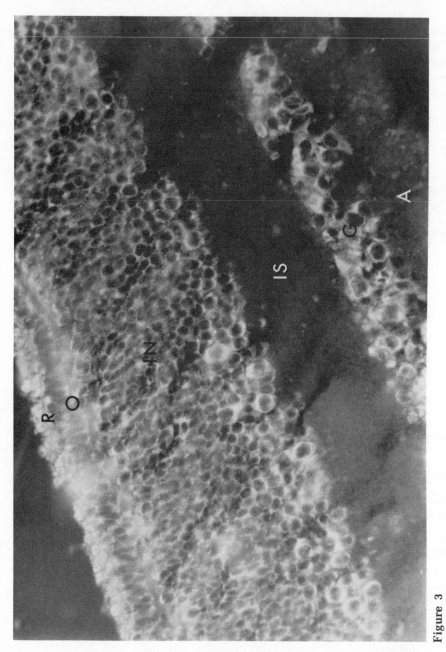

Figure 3

Antibody A2B5 labels cell bodies but not processes in sections of 16-day embryonic chick retina, as seen by indirect immunofluorescence. (R) Photoreceptor layer; (O) outer synaptic layer; (IN) inner nuclear layer; (IS) inner synaptic layer; (G) ganglion cell layer; (A) ganglion cell axons.

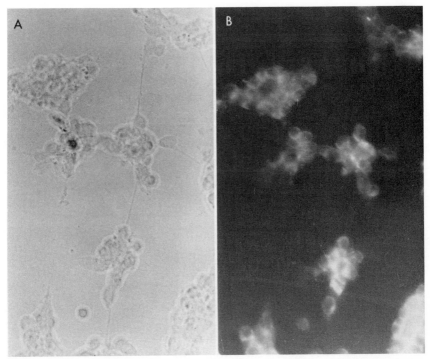

Figure 4
Distribution of antigen A2B5 on soma but not processes of chick embryo retina cells in short-term monolayer culture (8 days in ovo plus 1 day in vitro). (A) Phase-contrast view; (B) indirect immunofluorescence.

(NINCD, National Institutes of Health), inhibited A2B5 cytotoxicity with an ID_{50} of 0.2 μM. Crude bovine gangliosides and N-acetylneuraminic acid were also inhibitory, with half-maximal effects at 600 μM and 5000 μM, respectively. However, mono-, di-, and trisialogangliosides (GM_1, GD_1, and GT_1) and glucosaminic acid had no effect.

ANTIBODY A2B5 LABELS PEPTIDERGIC ENDOCRINE CELLS

• Because peptidergic endocrine cells, although conventionally regarded as derived from endoderm (Pictet et al. 1976), exhibit functional homologies with cells from the neural crest, a number of endocrine systems were tested for antigen A2B5. Using cryostat sections of adult rat pancreas, the antibody was found to label specifically islet cells but not acinar cells, which are exocrine (Fig. 6). Monolayer cultures of rat pancreatic cells revealed the antigen on the surface membranes of insulin-producing cells, by means of double-

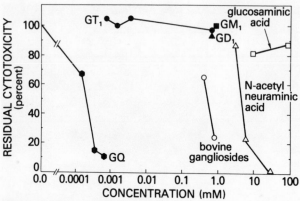

Figure 5

Inhibition of antibody A2B5—mediated complement-dependent cytotoxicity by defined ganglioside preparations and saccharides.

labeling techniques, but not on fibroblasts (Fig. 7). Highly purified populations of islet cells, free of acinar cells, have been obtained with the fluorescence-activated cell sorter (data not shown).

In the adrenal gland, the antigen was found on medullary cells but not on cortical cells (Fig. 8). Labeling was obtained with pituitary cells as well as with melanocytes, which are derived from the neural crest. Little or no antigen was found on cells from thyroid or testes.

Human tumors or cell lines that express antigen A2B5 include insulinomas, pheochromocytomas, medullary carcinoma of the thyroid, and melanomas, in addition to neuroblastomas.

The expression of antigen A2B5 was studied in greater detail in the rat insulinoma cell line RIN (Gazdar et al. 1980), derived from the transplantable RISL islet cell tumor of NEDH rats (Chick et al. 1977), and in its functionally distinct subclones. Antibody A2B5 labels both the parental RIN cells and the insulin-producing subclone RINm5F (Fig. 9). However, few, if any, cells in the subclone RINm14B, which secretes somatostatin, have levels of antigen detected by immunofluorescence.

A RAPID VISUAL ASSAY TO MONITOR PURIFICATION OF MEMBRANE ANTIGENS

• A technique was developed to facilitate purification of solubilized membrane antigens that react with monoclonal antibodies (Eisenbarth et al. 1980). Present methods for detecting soluble membrane antigens require specific classes of molecules (e.g., proteins with exposed

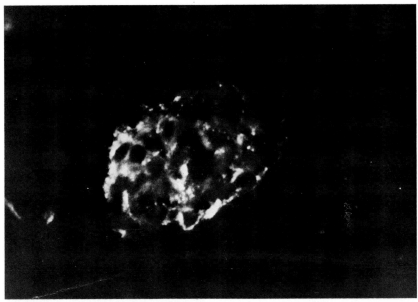

Figure 6
Localization of antigen A2B5 to islet cells, but not exocrine cells, in sections of neonatal rat pancreas, as seen by indirect immunofluorescence.

tyrosine residues for lactoperoxidase iodination) or are prohibited in the presence of requisite detergent concentrations to achieve solubilization (e.g., complement-dependent cytotoxicity). Polyvinyl chloride microtiter plates can be pretreated with a diluted monoclonal antibody, washed to remove unbound immunoglobulin, and then incubated with solubilized antigen: The antigen competitively inhibits the binding of target cells to immobilized antibody. In the absence of adsorbed antibody, or after antibody-sensitized wells are treated with antigen, target cells pellet to the bottom of the well upon centrifugation. In the absence of antigen, the immobilized antibody binds the target cells to the plastic as a diffuse mat, and no pellet forms. The visual microtiter assay was employed to monitor purification of the human-T-lymphocyte antigen 3A1, which designates a functionally distinct class of T cells (Haynes et al. 1979, 1980).

DISCUSSION

• Functional similarities among peptidergic endocrine cells and derivatives of neural crest and neural tube may be amenable to biochemical analysis through the use of monoclonal antibodies to shared

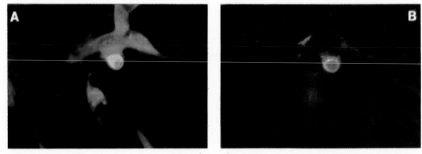

Figure 7. *(See facing page for legend.)*

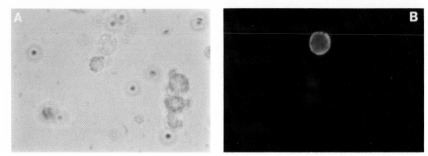

Figure 8. *(See facing page for legend.)*

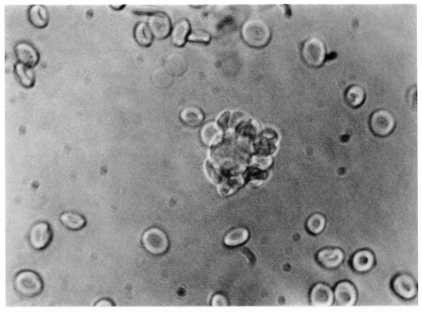

Figure 9. *(See facing page for legend.)*

surface-membrane molecules. Monoclonal antibodies are valuable reagents for identifying homologies as well as differences of cell type and for antigen isolation and characterization, with emphasis on (1) antibodies to functionally distinct clonal peptide-secreting cell lines and (2) rapid general methods for the purification of surface-membrane antigens of differentiated cells. As with neurons, the expression of receptors for antibody A2B5 by islet cells and other "APUD" (amine precursor uptake and decarboxylase) cells suggests that complex gangliosides are major membrane components of these cells.

REFERENCES

Chick, W.L., S. Warren, R.N. Chute, A.A. Like, V. Lauris, and K.C. Kitchen. 1977. A transplantable insulinoma in the rat. *Proc. Natl. Acad. Sci.* **74**:628.

Eisenbarth, G.S., F.S. Walsh, and M. Nirenberg. 1979. Monoclonal antibody to a plasma membrane antigen of neurons. *Proc. Natl. Acad. Sci.* **76**:4913.

Eisenbarth, G.S., R.B. Rankin, B.F. Haynes, and A.S. Fauci. 1980. A visual assay to monitor purification of cell surface antigens reacting with monoclonal antibodies. *J. Immunol. Methods* **39**:387.

Eisenbarth, G.S., H. Oie, A. Gazdar, W. Chick, J.A. Schultz, and R.M. Scearce. 1981. Production of monoclonal antibody reacting with rat islet cell membrane antigens. *Diabetes* **30**:226.

Galfre, G., S.C. Howe, C. Milstein, G.W. Butcher, and J.C. Howard. 1977. Antibodies to major histocompatibility antigens produced by hybrid cell lines. *Nature* **266**:550.

Gazdar, A.F., W.L. Chick, H.K. Oie, H.L. Sims, D.L. King, G.C. Weir, and V. Lauries. 1980. Continuous, clonal, insulin- and somatostatin-secreting cell lines established from a transplantable rat islet cell tumor. *Proc. Natl. Acad. Sci.* **77**:3523.

Haynes, B.F., G.S. Eisenbarth, and A.S. Fauci. 1979. Human lymphocyte antigens: Production of a monoclonal antibody that defines functional thymus-derived lymphocyte subsets. *Proc. Natl. Acad. Sci.* **76**:5829.

Figure 7
Indirect immunofluorescence of antigen A2B5 in monolayer cultures of rat pancreatic cells.

Figure 8
Indirect immunofluorescence of antigen A2B5 on adrenal medullary cells.

Figure 9
Detection of antibody A2B5 binding to RINm5F clonal rat insulinoma cells by protein A−treated erythrocytes.

Haynes, B.F., D.L. Mann, M.E. Helmer, J.A. Schroer, J.H. Shelhamer, G.S. Eisenbarth, J.L. Strominger, C.A. Thomas, H.S. Mostowski, and A.S. Fauci. 1980. Characterization of a monoclonal antibody that defines an immunoregulatory T-cell subset for immunoglobulin synthesis in humans. *Proc. Natl. Acad. Sci.* **77**:2914.

Ledeen, R.W. and R.K. Yu. 1978. Method for isolation and analysis of gangliosides. *Res. Methods Neurochem.* **4**:371.

Pictet, R.L., L.B. Rall, P. Phelps, and W.J. Rutter. 1976. The neural crest and the origin of the insulin-producing and other gastrointestinal hormone producing cells. *Science* **191**:191.

Schneider, M.D. and G.S. Eisenbarth, 1979. Transfer plate radioassay using cell monolayers to detect anti-cell-surface antibodies synthesized by lymphocyte hybridomas. *J. Immunol. Methods* **29**:331.

Developmental Studies of Rat Retina Cells Using Cell-type-specific Monoclonal Antibodies

COLIN J. BARNSTABLE

Department of Neurobiology
Harvard Medical School
Boston, Massachusetts 02115

• Differences among specific functional classes of neural cells are believed to be expressed, in part, by differences in cell-surface molecules (Sidman 1972; Moscona 1974; Rutishauser et al. 1978). As probes for membrane determinants limited to discrete subpopulations of neurons, anti-cell-surface antibodies have been of some use, but progress has been hindered by the vast heterogeneity of the immune response against available preparations of plasma membrane molecules (Fields et al. 1975; Schachner et al. 1976; Stallcup and Cohn 1976; Raff et al. 1979). Investigations of neuronal cell types, accordingly, have been facilitated by the production of monoclonal antibodies (Köhler and Milstein 1975; Barnstable 1980). The retina is a favorable model system in which to study surface markers that define different cell types because it (1) is readily accessible, (2) has only seven basic neural cell types, (3) generally allows assignment of cell type on the basis of position within a highly ordered laminar structure, and (4) has been amenable to physiological and biochemical studies of single dissociated cells.

INITIAL CHARACTERIZATION OF ANTIBODIES

• Female BALB/c mice were immunized intraperitoneally on days 0 and 21 with 200 μg of a crude membrane preparation of adult CD rat retina in complete Freund's adjuvant, and intravenously on day 42 with 100 μg of retina membrane protein in saline. On day 46, dissociated spleen cells were fused with either P3-NS1/1-Ag4-1 or 8653 mouse myeloma cells, and hybrid cell cultures were selected and

219

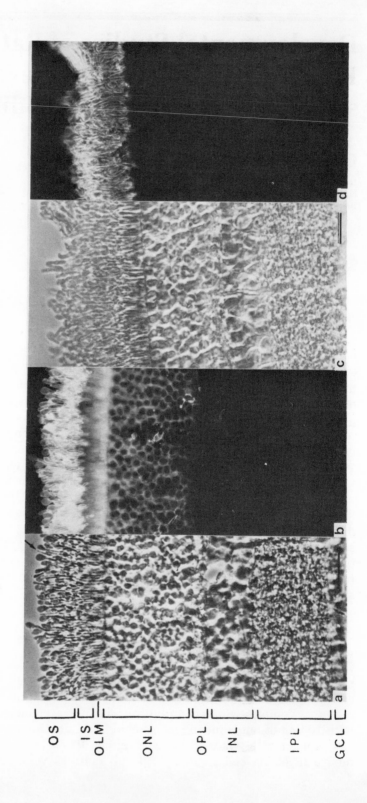

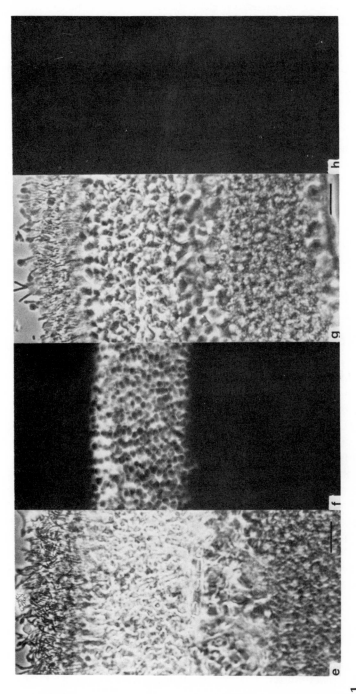

Figure 1
Indirect immunofluorescent labeling of sections of adult rat retina by antibodies RET-P1 (*a*, *b*), RET-P2 (*c*, *d*), and RET-P3 (*e*, *f*), employing rhodamine-conjugated goat anti–mouse IgG that had been affinity-purified on mouse IgG–Sepharose 4B. Sections (15 µm) were prepared on a freezing microtome using retinas that had been fixed with 1% paraformaldehyde, 0.1% glutaraldehyde for 1 hr, and treated with 30% (w/v) sucrose overnight. Nonspecific fluorescence (*g*, *h*) was determined using a monoclonal antibody against a human cell-surface glycoprotein as the primary antibody. (*a*, *c*, *e*, *g*) Phase-contrast and (*b*, *d*, *f*, *h*) epifluorescence micrographs are shown for each field. (OS) Outer segment; (IS) inner segment; (OLM) outer limiting membrane; (ONL) outer nuclear layer; (OPL) outer plexiform layer; (INL) inner nuclear layer; (IPL) inner plexiform layer; (GCL) ganglion cell layer. Scale bar, 20 µm.

221

cloned by standard techniques (Barnstable et al. 1978; Brodsky et al. 1979). Initial screening of hybridoma tissue culture supernatants comprised (1) an indirect radioimmunoassay employing adult rat retina that had been lightly homogenized and fixed with 0.5% paraformaldehyde as target particles, and (2) the $[^{125}I]F(ab')_2$ fragment of affinity-purified rabbit anti–mouse IgG to detect bound hybridoma antibodies. Antibodies selected for further characterization were unreactive with rat thymocytes or with cultured fibroblasts derived from neonatal rat lung. Tissue distribution of each antigen was then further tested by quantitative absorption of each antibody, respectively, with varying amounts of membrane from retina, cerebral cortex, cerebellum, or liver. The residual anti-retina antibody activity was then determined by $[^{125}I]F(ab')_2$ binding. Indirect immunofluorescent staining was performed on frozen sections of adult rat retina to establish the expression of each antigen by the individual subpopulations of retina cells.

THREE ANTIGENS LOCALIZED TO PHOTORECEPTORS

• Hybridoma antibody RET-P1 labeled the whole photoreceptor layer with ring fluorescence around almost all the photoreceptor cell bodies (Fig. 1). Whereas the photoreceptor inner segments were labeled at essentially the same intensity as the cell bodies, much brighter fluorescence was exhibited by photoreceptor outer segments. More-decisive evidence for restricted topographic distribution within the photoreceptor plasma membrane was seen with antibodies RET-P2 and RET-P3 (Fig. 1). Within the limitations of indirect immunofluorescence techniques, antibody RET-P2 labeled only the outer segments of photoreceptors, and antibody RET-P3 labeled only photoreceptor cell bodies. These differential labeling patterns seen with three monoclonal antibodies specific for photoreceptors suggest that some photoreceptor membrane molecules are common to all regions of the cell, whereas others are restricted to discrete regions of the cell. The molecular mechanisms for this differential localization of antigen are unclear at present, but they include localized insertion of newly synthesized molecules into a nonfluid domain of plasma membrane and anchorage of particular molecules to cytoskeletal or extracellular elements.

Because the rat retina consists almost entirely of rods (La Vail 1976), it was impossible to ascertain with this species whether these antibodies were reactive with cones as well. RET-P2 and RET-P3 appeared, however, to be rat-specific, whereas the RET-P1 antigenic determinant was found to be present in photoreceptors of many species, including rat, mouse, rabbit, turtle, tiger salamander, and goldfish. In the tiger salamander (*Ambystoma tigrinum*), antigen RET-P1 was found on rods but not on adjacent cones (Fig. 2).

SIX ANTIBODIES SPECIFICALLY LABEL MÜLLER CELLS

• Müller cells, the glial cells of the retina, have a unique morphology in that they are the only retinal cell type to extend radially across the retina from the outer limiting membrane to the inner limiting membrane. Six antibodies were found that label the essential features of their structure (Fig. 3), i.e., fine, fingerlike processes that extend up between the inner halves of photoreceptor inner segments; thick, radial Müller fibers passing through the outer nuclear layer; three bands of tangential labeling in the inner plexiform layer; and bulbous feet that surround the ganglion cell layer.

As a further test of cell-type specificity, one of the antibodies, RET-G1, was tested by indirect immunofluorescence of enzymatically dissociated cells from adult rat retina (Fig. 4). Only cells with the morphology of Müller cells were labeled. Antibody RET-G1 also

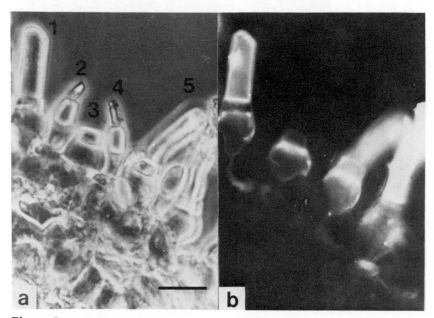

Figure 2
(a) Phase-contrast and (b) epifluorescence micrographs of tiger salamander photoreceptors labeled by antibody RET-P1 as described in the legend to Fig. 1. Cells labeled 1, 3, and 5 are rods, and cells 2 and 4 are cones. Scale bar, 20 μm.

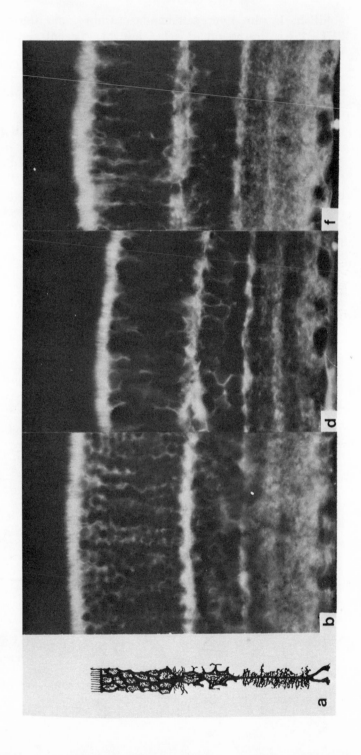

224

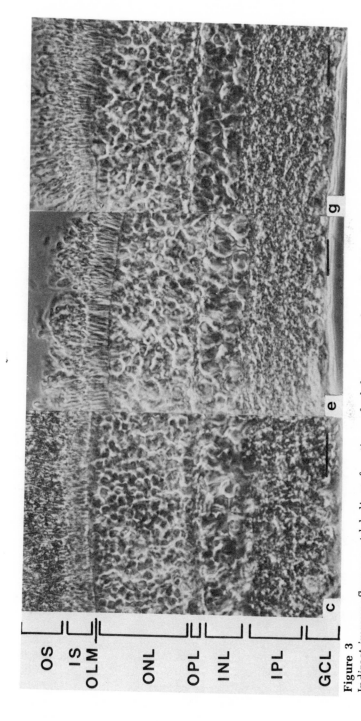

Figure 3

Indirect immunofluorescent labeling of sections of adult rat retina by antibodies RET-G1 (*b, c*), RET-G2 (*d, e*), and RET-G3 (*f, g*). Epifluorescence (*b, d, f*) and phase-contrast (*c, e, g*) micrographs are shown for each field. (*a*) A Müller cell of Golgi-stained retina as drawn by Santiago Ramon y Cajal (1955). (OS) Outer segment; (IS) inner segment; (OLM) outer limiting membrane; (ONL) outer nuclear layer; (OPL) outer plexiform layer; (INL) inner nuclear layer; (IPL) inner plexiform layer; (GCL) ganglion cell layer. Scale bar, 20 μm.

225

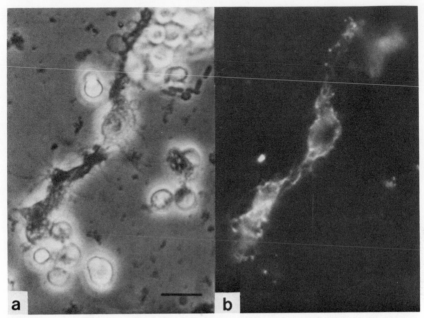

Figure 4
(a) Phase-contrast and (b) epifluorescence micrographs of enzymatically dissociated Müller cells labeled by antibody RET-G1. Scale bar, 10 μm.

reacted with glial cells in adult rat cerebral cortex and all layers of cerebellum, whereas none of the other five antibodies that specifically label retina Müller cells reacted with glia in other regions of the central nervous system. This result was confirmed by absorption analysis, which showed that RET-G1, but not the other five antibodies against glial cells, was absorbed by cerebral cortex and cerebellum membranes. These results emphasize both the similarities of and the differences between Müller cells and glia elsewhere in the central nervous system.

A NEURON-SPECIFIC ANTIGEN OF THE RETINA AND THE CENTRAL NERVOUS SYSTEM

• Antibody RET-N1 labeled most, if not all, of the neuronal cells in adult rat retina (Fig. 5). The antigen was found on the photoreceptor inner segments, both plexiform layers, many cell bodies in the outer half of the inner nuclear layer, axons of bipolar cells, and ganglion cells. No labeling characteristic of Müller cells was seen. The antibody additionally labels cells at all levels of cerebral cortex, and several cell types in the cerebellum (Fig. 5b), although in a pattern different from that given by antibody RET-G1 (Fig. 5c). Testing of antibodies RET-G1 and RET-N1 against glia and neurons, respectively, of the peripheral nervous system is in progress.

PRELIMINARY BIOCHEMICAL CHARACTERIZATION

• Antigens RET-P1 and RET-P2 copurify with retina plasma membranes in differential and sucrose density gradient centrifugation, are resistant to heating at 100°C for 10 minutes, and are soluble in both 2% NP-40 or 2% deoxycholate. RET-G1 and RET-N1 antigens are insoluble under these conditions of detergent extraction and are resistant to trypsin, papain, or pronase.

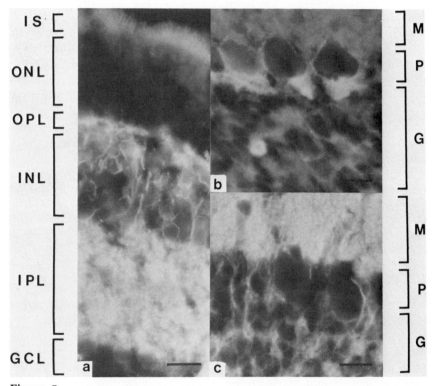

Figure 5
(a) Indirect immunofluorescent labeling of sectioned adult rat retina by antibody RET-N1. Indirect immunofluorescent labeling of sections of adult rat cerebellum by antibodies RET-N1 (b) and RET-G1 (c). (IS) Inner segment; (ONL) outer nuclear layer; (OPL) outer plexiform layer; (INL) inner nuclear layer; (IPL) inner plexiform layer; (GCL) ganglion cell layer; (M) molecular layer; (P) Purkinje cell layer; (G) granular layer. Scale bar, 20 μm.

EFFECT OF DEVELOPMENTAL AGE ON RETINAL ANTIGEN EXPRESSION

• Each of the three antigens localized specifically to photoreceptors is first detectable at a different developmental stage. RET-P1 antigen is first detectable at birth, on a small population (1%) of cells on the ventricular side of the developing retina. Each cell is bipolar, sending one process outward into the mid-portion of the retina and another inward to the ventricular surface, where it terminates in an intensely labeled structure that may correspond to the primary cilium of developing photoreceptors (Fig. 6). The number of cells in this layer that bear the RET-P1 antigen increases progressively with age. A relationship has yet to be established between antigen expression and withdrawal of photoreceptors from mitosis. RET-P2 antigen first appears in developing photoreceptor outer segments at day 5, the time of initial outer segment formation, shortly before the appearance of detectable opsin. RET-P3 antigen is not detected until day 12, just prior to eye opening. Thus, the antigens are markers not only of adult cell type, but also of precursor cells during neuronal maturation.

Three discrete developmental stages are also characteristic of the Müller-cell-specific antigens. RET-G1 is present at birth, RET-G2 appears at day 7, and the other four antigens do not appear until days 12–14.

Initial experiments have shown that RET-P1 and RET-G2 are also expressed by monolayer cultures of retina cells prepared with cells from retinae of varying ages. However, the morphology of cells in vitro does not invariably follow the in vivo pattern: In culture, photoreceptor precursors detected by antibody RET-P1 were spherical and had only a single process, containing large varicosities.

DISCUSSION

• These investigations clearly demonstrate that monoclonal antibodies can be produced that recognize specific functional subpopulations of the mammalian central nervous system and indicate a number of the potential uses for these reagents. The expression of these molecules on dissociated cells facilitates their use as markers for selective enrichment or depletion of cell types by fluorescence-activated cell sorting or complement-mediated cytotoxicity in order to prepare defined cell classes for developmental, physiological, and biochemical studies. The developmental regulation observed with these antigens makes possible the detailed study of in vivo and in vitro maturation of single cell types along with simple, quantitative assays for modulators of the differentiation process. Finally, mono-

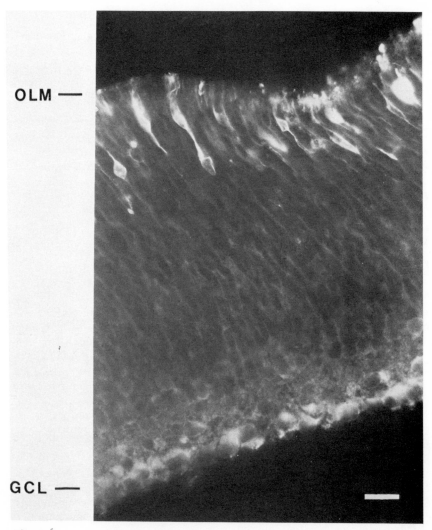

Figure 6
Indirect immunofluorescent labeling of sectioned retina from 2-day-old rat by
antibody RET-P1. (OLM) Outer limiting membrane; (GCL) ganglion cell layer.
Scale bar, 20 μm.

clonal antibodies can be used to elucidate the nature and function of
surface membrane molecules that are restricted by cell type or by
region within the plasma membrane of single cells, so as to facilitate
an understanding of the molecular and genetic basis of neural structure and function.

REFERENCES

Barnstable, C.J. 1980. Monoclonal antibodies which recognise different cell types in the rat retina. *Nature* **286**:231.

Barnstable, C.J., W.F. Bodmer, G. Brown, G. Galfre, C. Milstein, A.F. Williams, and A. Ziegler. 1978. Production of monoclonal antibodies to group A erythrocytes, HLA and other human cell surface antigens—New tools for genetic analysis. *Cell* **14**:9.

Brodsky, F.M., P. Parham, C.J. Barnstable, M.J. Crumpton, and W.F. Bodmer. 1979. Monoclonal antibodies for analysis of the HLA system. *Immunol. Rev.* **47**:3.

Cajal, S.R. 1955. *Histologie du systeme nerveux de l'homme et des vertebres,* vol. II. CSIC, Madrid.

Fields, K.L., C. Gosling, M. Megson, and P.L. Stern. 1975. New cell surface antigens in rat defined by tumors of the nervous system. *Proc. Natl. Acad. Sci.* **72**:1296.

Köhler, G. and C. Milstein. 1975. Continuous cultures of fused cells secreting antibody of predefined specificity. *Nature* **256**:495.

La Vail, M.M. 1976. Survival of some photoreceptor cells in albino rats following long-term exposure to continuous light. *Invest. Ophthal.* **15**: 64.

Moscona, A.A., ed. 1976. *The cell surface in development.* Wiley, New York.

Raff, M.C., K.L. Fields, S. Hakomori, R. Mirsky, R.M. Pruss, and J. Winter. 1979. Cell-type-specific markers for distinguishing and studying neurons and the major classes of glial cells in culture. *Brain Res.* **174**:283.

Rutishauser, V., R. Brackenbury, J.-P. Thiery, and G.M. Edelman. 1978. Cell-adhesion molecules from neural tissues of the chick embryo. *Birth defects: Original article series* **XIV**:305.

Schachner, M., M.Z. Ruberg, and T.B. Carnow. 1976. Histological localisation of nervous system antigens in the cerebellum by immunoperoxidase labelling. *Brain Res. Bull.* **1**:367.

Sidman, R.L. 1972. Cell interactions in developing mammalian central nervous system. In *Cell interactions* (ed. L.G. Silvestri), p. 1. North Holland, Amsterdam.

Stallcup, W.B. and M. Cohn. 1976. Correlation of surface antigens and cell type in cloned cell lines from the rat central nervous system. *Exp. Cell Res.* **98**:285.

A Gradient of Molecules in Avian Retina with Dorsoventral Polarity

G. DAVID TRISLER, MICHAEL D. SCHNEIDER, JOSEPH R. MOSKAL, and MARSHALL NIRENBERG

Laboratory of Biochemical Genetics
National Heart, Lung, and Blood Institute
National Institutes of Health
Bethesda, Maryland 20205

• Mechanisms that impart positional information for the assembly of the developing nervous system and the establishment of specific synaptic connections have been studied in model systems. The retina is a highly ordered laminar structure due to segregation of different classes of neuronal cell bodies and synapses into separate strata (Karten, this volume). Synaptic connections between retina ganglion neurons and tectum neurons preserve the topographic relations of ganglion neurons in the retina, resulting in a point-to-point retino-tectal map. However, the mechanisms underlying these phenomena have not been defined. Sperry (1963) postulated that two orthogonal gradients of molecules on retina ganglion neurons and corresponding gradients of complementary molecules in the optic tectum might determine the specificity of connections between retina and tectum neurons. Other mechanisms that have been proposed include adhesive interactions between migrating retina neurites, myelination of bundles of retina axons, and formation of extracellular channels by glia to guide retina axons (Silver and Sidman 1980).

Antisera have been widely used to study retinal structure and function (Goldschneider and Moscona 1972; Thiery et al. 1977; Hausman and Moscona 1979). Clonal neural retina hybrid cell lines derived from single retina cells (as a homogeneous immunogen) have been used to produce rabbit antiserum demonstrating an antigen of the rodent neural retina that was expressed in a restricted topographic domain (Trisler et al. 1979). Hybridoma cell lines were derived by fusing mouse myeloma cells with spleen cells from mice immunized with retina cells to produce monoclonal antibodies to retina neurons or Müller cells (Eisenbarth et al. 1979; Barnstable 1980).

To detect cell-surface molecules with topographic specificity in the retina, hybridoma antibodies, as candidates for neuronal recognition molecules, were obtained by fusing P3-X63/Ag-8 mouse myeloma cells (Köhler and Milstein 1975) with spleen cells from mice immunized with small portions of dorsal or ventral 14-day chick embryo neural retina or clonal retina hybrid cells. A hybridoma antibody was obtained that binds to cell-membrane molecules distributed in a dorsoposterior → ventroanterior gradient in retina (Trisler et al. 1981).

DETECTION OF ANTIBODIES WITH TOPOGRAPHIC SPECIFICITY

• The rationale for the experiments shown schematically in Figure 1 was to immunize mice with cells from dorsoposterior or ventral 14-day chick embryo left retina to obtain hybridoma cell lines synthesizing antibody with specificity for the retina sector used for immunization. The choroid fissure was used as a landmark. Female BALB/c

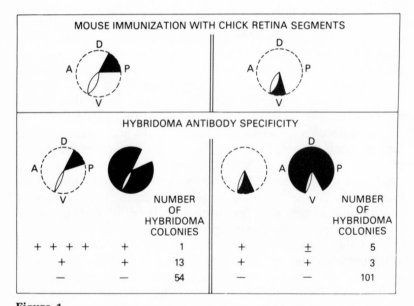

Figure 1
Strategy for detecting region-specific retina surface-membrane antigens. Lymphocyte hybridomas were derived from mice immunized with cells from dorsoposterior (*left panels*) or ventral (*right panels*) retina; hybridoma antibody binding to paired cultured-cell monolayers from the portions of 14-day chick embryo retina shown in black in the lower panels was determined.

mice were immunized on days 0, 7, and 14 intraperitoneally with 8×10^6 mechanically dissociated retina cells and intravenously with 2×10^6 cells from dorsoposterior or ventral retina. On the 17th day, 1×10^8 spleen cells from an immunized mouse were fused with 2×10^7 P3-X63/Ag-8 mouse myeloma cells as described by Galfre et al. (1977). After fusion, the cells were suspended with 5×10^6 spleen cells from a nonimmunized mouse in 50 ml of medium (Trisler et al. 1981), and 672 wells of 96-well microculture plates were inoculated with cells (74 μl/well). Additional medium was added (0.1 ml/well) on the 5th and 10th days after fusion.

To detect an antibody to a surface molecule enriched in one region of the retina, tissue culture supernatants from wells with hybridoma colonies were tested by indirect radioimmunoassay against cells cultured for 2 days (Schneider and Eisenbarth 1979);

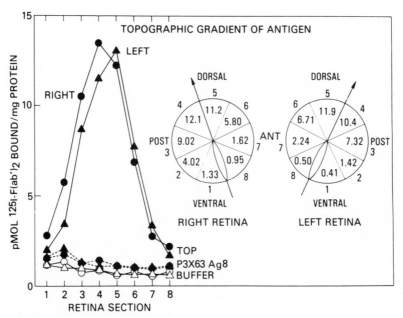

Figure 2

Topographic gradient of TOP antigen in ($\bullet$) right or ($\blacktriangle$) left 14-day chick embryo neural retina. Equivalent sectors from different retinas were pooled and assayed for $[^{125}I]F(ab')_2$ binding after incubation with ($\bullet$————$\bullet$; $\blacktriangle$————$\blacktriangle$) TOP antibody, ($\bullet$--------$\bullet$; $\blacktriangle$--------$\blacktriangle$) P3-X63/Ag-8 antibody, or ($\circ$————$\circ$, $\triangle$————$\triangle$) buffer in the absence of antibody. The right half of the figure depicts, within each sector of the retina, the pmoles of specifically bound $[^{125}I]F(ab')_2$ per mg of retina protein (binding due to antibody to TOP minus binding due to antibody synthesized by P3-X63/Ag-8 parental cells). Assay conditions are described in the legend to Fig. 3.

cells were taken from the one eighth of the retina originally used as immunogen or from the remaining seven eighths of the retina. Hybridoma antibody binding to retina cells was detected with an ^{125}I-labeled, affinity-purified $F(ab')_2$ fragment of rabbit anti—mouse IgG ($[^{125}I]F(ab')_2$).

A TOPOGRAPHIC GRADIENT OF SURFACE-MEMBRANE MOLECULES

• One of 155 hybridoma cell lines examined synthesized antibody to a cell-surface antigen distributed preferentially in dorsoposterior retina (Fig. 2), designated TOP, for toponymic antigen (i.e., a marker of position). Neural retinas from right or left eyes of 14-day chick

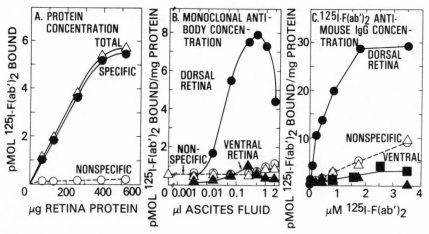

Figure 3
(A) Effect of dorsal retina protein concentration (pooled sections 4 and 5 from 14-day chick embryos as illustrated in Fig. 2) on $[^{125}I]F(ab')_2$ binding due to: (Δ) antibody to TOP; (o) antibody synthesized by P3-X63/Ag-8; (•) specific binding. (B) Effect of monoclonal antibody concentration on (•, ▲) $[^{125}I]F(ab')_2$ specific binding due to antibody to TOP or (o, Δ) nonspecific binding due to P3-X63/Ag-8 antibody, to cells from (•) dorsal retina sections 4 and 5 or (▲) ventral retina sections 1 and 8. (C) Effect of concentration of $[^{125}I]F(ab')_2$ rabbit anti—mouse IgG. For all experiments each reaction mixture contained the following components, except where specified, in a final volume of 50 μl: 150—200 μg of retina protein, 50 μg of gelatin, and 1 μl of hybridoma ascites fluid; the reaction mixtures were incubated for 30 min at 4°C and washed three times. The pellets were resuspended in 50 μl containing 440 nM $[^{125}I]F(ab')_2$ (50,000 cpm), 50 μg of gelatin, and 500 μg of bovine serum albumin in Dulbecco's phosphate-buffered saline, incubated for 30 min at 4°C, washed three times, and counted.

embryos were cut into eight 45° sectors and assayed for TOP antigen. The highest concentration of antigen detected was in dorsoposterior retina and the lowest in ventroanterior retina. Bilaterally symmetric gradients were found in right and left eyes. Other hybridoma antibodies, including A2B5 (Eisenbarth et al. 1979), bound equally to cells from each region of retina.

The effects of varying concentrations of retina protein, hybridoma antibody, and [^{125}I]F(ab')$_2$ rabbit anti–mouse IgG are shown in Figure 3, A, B, and C, respectively. Assay conditions employed are summarized in the legend to Figure 3.

To determine whether the TOP antigen gradient is polar (i.e., varies with angle of rotation around the center of the retina), with

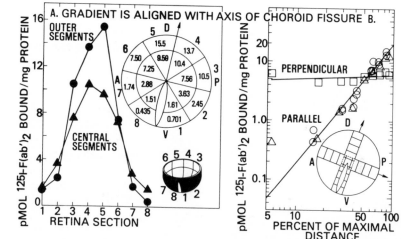

Figure 4

Orientation of the TOP gradient. Specific binding of [^{125}I]F(ab')$_2$ (pmoles per mg of protein) is shown within the appropriate segment of retina in A and on the ordinate in A and B. (A) Each left retina was cut into eight 45° sectors (7.25 mm in length), which were divided into central (4.9 mm) and outer (2.35 mm) segments. (B) Demonstration that TOP concentration detected is a function of the square of distance from the ventroanterior margin of the retina. (Δ) Strips of retina 2.5 mm wide running from the ventroanterior margin (0% distance) to the dorsoposterior margin of the retina (14.5 mm = 100% of maximal distance), parallel to the choroid fissure, were removed from eight retinas (left eyes) and each was cut into nine 1.5-mm segments as shown. (□) Strips of retina from anterior (0%) to posterior (100%) margins of retina were prepared and assayed as above. (o) The data from A. The length of the arc from the ventral pole of the gradient to the center of each segment was calculated assuming the retina to be a hemisphere and using equations relating angles and sides of spherical triangles.

uniform antigen concentration along any line of radius, or varies with distance from the dorsoposterior to the ventroanterior margins of the retina, left retinas of 14-day chick embryos were divided into 16 sections as shown in Figure 4A and assayed for TOP. Specific $[^{125}I]F(ab')_2$ binding varied from 0.35 pmoles per mg of protein at the ventroanterior margin to 15.5 pmoles per mg of protein at the dorsoposterior margin of the retina. Thus, a 35-fold gradient of TOP antigen was detected, aligned with the dorsoposterior-ventroanterior axis of the eye (i.e., oriented parallel to the long axis of the choroid fissure).

Antigen concentration detected was a logarithmic function of distance from the dorsoposterior pole of the gradient to the ventroanterior pole along the circumference of the retina (Fig. 4B). In contrast, little or no variation in TOP antigen concentration was detected along the axis perpendicular to the choroid fissure. The concentration of $[^{125}I]F(ab')_2 \cdot$anti-TOP antibody$\cdot$TOP antigen complex detected (F_x) is a function of the square of the circumferential distance (D_x) from the ventroanterior pole of the gradient toward the dorsoposterior pole. Thus, TOP molecules can be used as a marker of cell position along a ventroanterior-dorsoposterior axis of retina, i.e.,

$$D_x = D_{max} (F_x/F_{max})^{0.5},$$

where D_{max} and F_{max} are maximal values for retina at the dorsoposterior margin of the retina. Under the conditions used for the experiments shown in Figure 4, A and B, F_{max} was 20 pmoles of $[^{125}I]F(ab')_2$ bound specifically per mg of protein, and D_{max} was 14.5 mm. Thus, the calculated mean position in retina of cells that bind 5 pmoles of $[^{125}I]F(ab')_2$ specifically per mg of protein is 7.25 mm from the ventroanterior pole of the gradient, which agrees well with the experimentally determined values.

EXPRESSION OF TOP ANTIGEN DURING DEVELOPMENT

• The antigen was detected in the optic cups of 48-hour chick embryos, and evidence for a gradient of TOP in retina was found with 4-day chick embryos, the earliest stage tested, through the adult (Fig. 5). Whereas the amount of TOP detected per mg of ventral retina protein remained constant throughout development, the concentration of TOP antigen in dorsal retina increased threefold between the 4th and 12th days of embryonic development and then decreased somewhat in the adult. In summary, these results suggest that a gradient of TOP molecules is formed early in retina development, during active neuroblast proliferation and neuron genesis, and is maintained after neuron genesis ceases.

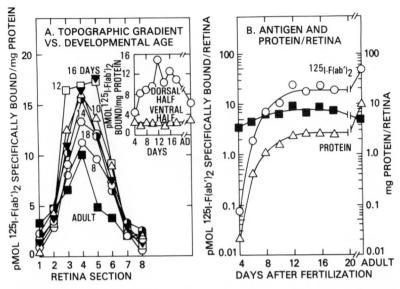

Figure 5
Expression of TOP antigen in chick retina during embryonic development and in the adult. (A) Symbols represent antigen concentration
detected in each of eight radial sectors of retina (shown in Fig. 2) from
chick embryos at: (o) day 8, (Δ) 10, (□) 12, (◐) 14, (▼) 16, (◑) 18, and
(■) adult. The insert depicts antigen detected in dorsal or ventral halves
of retina from 4- through 18-day embryos and adults. (B) (o) TOP
antigen detected per retina; (Δ) protein per retina; (■) [^{125}I]F(ab')$_2$ specifically bound per mg of protein.

A chick embryo was found with a third eye in the middle of the
forehead (Fig. 6); retinas from the right, middle, and left eyes each
had a gradient of TOP molecules with normal symmetry, polarity, and
orientation. Thus, a gradient of TOP with normal orientation was
generated in the third eye despite the abnormal orientation of the eye
in the embryo.

ANTIGEN DISTRIBUTION

• The antigen was detected by autoradiography (Fig. 7) or indirect
immunofluorescence on most, if not all, cell types in 14-day chick
embryo dorsoposterior retina. More antigen was detected in the inner
and outer synaptic regions than elsewhere in the retina. Little antigen
was detected in ventroanterior retina. All mechanically dissociated
cells examined from 8-day chick embryo dorsoposterior retina had
punctate rim fluorescence; all cells examined from middle retina also

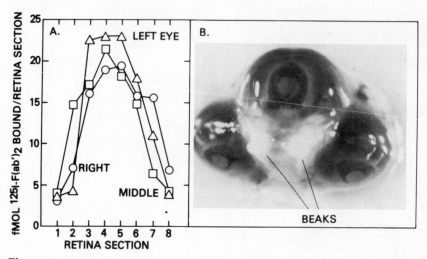

Figure 6

(A) TOP antigen gradients in retinas from the (o) right, (□) middle, and (Δ) left eyes of a 14-day chick embryo with three eyes. Total $[^{125}I]F(ab')_2$ bound per retina section is shown. Reaction mixtures contained 2.38 nM $[^{125}I]F(ab')_2$. (B) Frontal view of head of embryo. The third eye is situated on the forehead and oriented in a dorsoanterior direction. The embryo had two pairs of beaks, two brains in one head, and one body.

were fluorescent, but less intensely than dorsoposterior retina cells. No fluorescent cells were detected in ventroanterior retina.

The highest concentrations of TOP antigen were found in tissue derived from the forebrain (Table 1): retina > cerebrum > thalamus. Lower levels of antigen were found in optic nerve, cerebellum, dorsal and ventral retina pigment epithelium, and optic tectum. Little or no antigen was detected in heart, liver, kidney, or blood cells.

Gradients of TOP molecules with similar orientation and symmetry were detected in turkey, quail, and duck retina (Fig. 8), but the antigen was not detected in goldfish, *Xenopus laevis*, *Rana pipiens*, or postnatal Fisher rat retina.

PROPERTIES OF TOP ANTIGEN

• Incubation of 14-day chick embryo retina cells at 100°C or incubation at 37°C with 11 μM trypsin resulted in loss of antigenic activity from cells (Table 2). To study the possible involvement of carbohydrate residues, hapten-competition experiments were performed (Table 2). Incubation of retina cells with wheat germ agglutinin (which binds to β-N-acetylglucosaminyl residues) at 4°C reduced

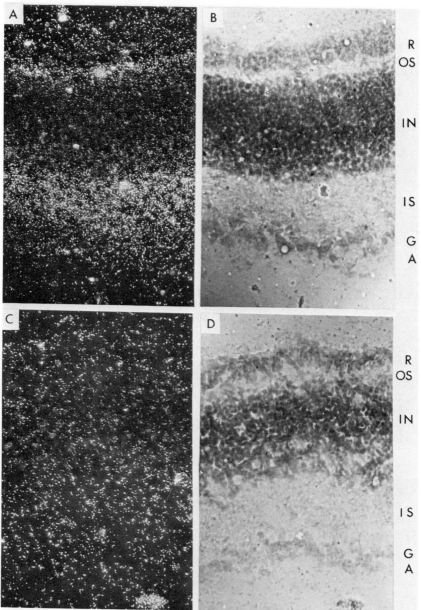

Figure 7

Autoradiographs of 14-day chick embryo retina. Frozen sections (16 μm) from outer halves of dorsal or ventral retina were treated with antibody to TOP, followed by [^{125}I]F(ab')$_2$, exposed 22 days, and stained with toluidine blue. (A) Dark-field and (B) phase-contrast views of dorsal retina. In A, some silver grains over cell soma in the inner nuclear layer appear dim due to staining of cells by toluidine blue. (C) Dark-field and (D) phase-contrast views of ventral retina. (R) photoreceptor layer; (OS) outer synaptic layer; (IN) inner nuclear layer; (IS) inner synaptic layer; (G) ganglion cell layer; (A) ganglion cell axon layer. Magnification, 517×.

Table 1

Distribution of TOP Antigen in Chicken Tissues

Tissue	14-Day embryo	Adult
	(pmoles $[^{125}I]F(ab')_2$ specifically bound/mg protein)	
Dorsal neural retina	12.0	7.70
Ventral neural retina	1.08	2.70
Cerebrum	3.30	3.12
Thalamus	2.13	—
Optic nerve	—	0.58
Optic tectum	0.15	—
Cerebellum	0.23	0.46
Dorsal retina pigment epithelium	0.26	—
Ventral retina pigment epithelium	0.25	—
Heart, liver, kidney, or blood cells	0.002–0.055	

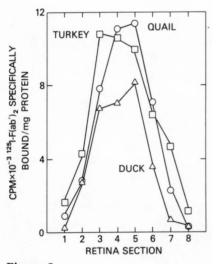

Figure 8

TOP antigen gradients in retina from:
(o) Japanese quail (15-day embryo);
(Δ) White Pekin duck (16-day embryo); (□) turkey (17-day embryo); the
eggs hatch 17, 28, and 28 days after
fertilization, respectively. $[^{125}I]F(ab')_2$
concentrations and μCi/pmole were
0.26 nM (0.90 μCi/pmole), 0.074 nM
(2.92 μCi/pmole), and 0.078 nM (2.38
μCi/pmole), respectively.

Table 2
Effect of Trypsin, Heat, or Lectins on TOP Antigenicity

Exp. no.	Treatment of retina cells		cpm [^{125}I]F(ab')$_2$ bound specifically to retina cells	%
	0–30 min	30–40 min		
1	control	+ trypsin inhibitor	1700	100
	trypsin	+ trypsin inhibitor	93	6
	trypsin + trypsin inhibitor	—	1803	106
2	4°C, 30 min		1607	100
	100°C, 30 min		132	8
3	control		467	100
	50 μg wheat germ agglutinin		271	58
	50 μg concanavalin A		951	204
	50 μg Ulex europaeus agglutinin I		607	130

Properties of TOP antigen molecules in 14-day chick embryo dorsal retina. In experiment 1, retina cells were incubated for 30 min at 37°C, in either phosphate-buffered saline (PBS), PBS with 11 μM trypsin (crystallized three times; Worthington), or PBS with 11 μM trypsin inactivated with 12 μM soybean trypsin inhibitor (Worthington), then for 10 min with soybean trypsin inhibitor. TOP ascites fluid was diluted 1000-fold; 1.86 nM [^{125}I]F(ab')$_2$ (9.05 × 10^{-2} μCi/pmole) was used. In experiment 2, TOP and P3-X63/Ag-8 antibodies were diluted 100-fold; 1.82 nM [^{125}I]F(ab')$_2$ (9.69 × 10^{-2} μCi/pmole) was used. In experiment 3, retina cells were incubated with lectins (50 μg per 6 × 10^6 cells) for 15 min at 4°C, washed to remove unbound lectin, and assayed for TOP. TOP and P3-X63/Ag-8 antibodies were diluted 500-fold.

antibody binding to 58% of the control value, whereas *Ulex europaeus* agglutinin I (specific for L-fucosyl residues) had no effect, and concanavalin A (specific for α-D-mannosyl and α-D-glucosyl residues) increased antibody binding twofold. Increased anti-TOP antibody binding was also observed after treatment with succinylated concanavalin A.

ANTIGEN CONTENT OF CULTURED RETINA CELLS

• Cells dissociated from 8-day chick embryo retina with 0.05% trypsin (crystallized three times), 0.003% collagenase, 2% chick serum, and 0.001% DNase contain little or no TOP antigen; however, cells cultured for 24 hours in vitro bound 50% as much antibody to TOP as did cells from intact retina in ovo. With cells dissociated with trypsin from dorsal or ventral 8-day embryo retina and cultured for 6 days, approximately the same amount of antigen per mg of protein was

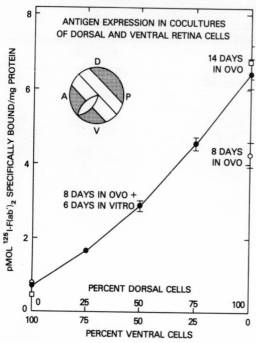

Figure 9

TOP antigen in monolayer cultures containing varying proportions of cells dissociated with 0.05% trypsin and 0.005% DNase from dorsal or ventral 8-day chick embryo retina and cultured for 6 days. Each 100-mm culture plate contained 8×10^7 retina cells and 15 ml of medium (90% Eagle's minimal essential medium, 10% fetal bovine serum).

detected as with dorsal and ventral 14-day chick embryo retina in ovo (Fig. 9). With trypsinized cells from dorsal and ventral retina that were mixed in different proportions and cocultured for 6 days, antigen levels detected were nearly additive (Fig. 9; linear correlation coefficient, r^2, 0.98). No evidence of induction or suppression of antigen was obtained under the conditions tested. Dorsal, middle, and ventral 8-day chick embryo retina cells were dissociated with trypsin collagenase, chick serum, and DNase, then cultured for 4 days, dissociated a second time by the same method, and cultured for 6 additional days. The antigen contents detected were similar to those found with dorsal, middle, and ventral retina cells that were dissociated only once and then were cultured for 10 days (Fig. 10). Thus, a gradient of antigen can be reexpressed and maintained for at least 10 days in culture.

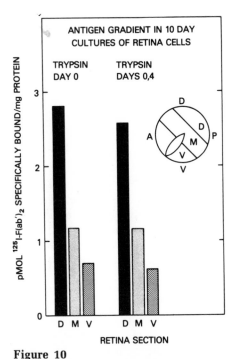

Figure 10
TOP antigen in monolayer cultures containing cells dissociated with 0.05%
trypsin, 0.003% collagenase, 2% chick
serum, and 0.001% DNase from dorsal,
middle, or ventral 8-day chick embryo
retina, and cultured for 10 days as in
Fig. 9; where indicated, cells were dissociated again as above on the 4th day
of culture, recovered, and cultured in
fresh 100-mm plates for 6 additional
days.

MONOCLONAL ANTIBODIES TO RETINA HYBRID CELL LINES

• As an alternative strategy to identify surface membrane molecules
localized to restricted topographic regions of the neural retina, monoclonal antibodies were generated against clonal hybrid cell lines
originated by fusing retina cells from rat, mouse, or Chinese hamster
embryos with clonal mouse neuroblastoma N18TG2 or human fibroblast VA-2-M7 cells. The retina hybrid cell lines used for immunization of mice were: NCE-9AK (Chinese hamster embryo retina ×
N18TG-2), N18RE-103 (Fisher rat embryo retina × N18TG-2), N18ME-
1 (C57/B1 mouse embryo retina × N18TG-2), and CHEM7A2al (Chinese hamster embryo retina × VA-2-M7). NCE-9AK, N18RE-103, and

N18ME-1 hybrid cells generate action potentials when stimulated electrically, possess tetrodotoxin-sensitive Na^+ channels, extend long neurites, and resemble neurons in morphology. N18RE-103 cells synthesize dopamine, and N18ME-1 cells synthesize norepinephrine (E. Heldman et al., unpubl.). In contrast, neither catecholamine synthesis nor tyrosine hydroxylase activity was detected in parental N18TG-2 neuroblastoma cells. NCE-9AK cells possess large, dense-core vesicles and are more adhesive to 10-day chick embryo retina cells than to cerebral cortex cells or N18TG-2 cells (M. Delong and M. Nirenberg, unpubl.).

Spleen cells from immunized mice were fused with P3-X63/Ag-8 mouse myeloma cells, and 1136 hybridoma cell lines were obtained; 133 hybridoma cell lines were obtained that synthesize antibodies that bind to the retina hybrid cells used for immunization (11.7%). Twenty-eight antibodies bound to retina hybrid cells but not to N18TG-2 or VA-2-M7 parental cells or other nonneural cell lines tested from the same species as the retina parental cells.

CONCLUSIONS

• A monoclonal antibody was obtained that defines a cell-surface antigen distributed in a 35-fold concentration gradient in avian retina. The concentration of antigen is highest at the dorsoposterior margin of the retina and lowest at the ventroanterior margin. The antigen was found on most or all cell types in chick retina, and the amount of antigen detected is related to cell position in the retina. The concentration of antigen found is a function of the square of circumferential distance from the ventroanterior pole of the gradient toward the dorsoposterior pole. The dorsoposterior portion of the retina differs from other portions of the retina in neuronal lineage and embryologic development, migration of cells and axons across the midline of the embryo, synapse specificity, adhesive specificity, and function. The function of TOP molecules has not been determined; however, our working hypothesis is that TOP molecules play a role in the encoding or decoding of positional information in the retina. The mechanism of generating and maintaining the highly ordered topographic gradient also remains to be determined.

REFERENCES

Barnstable, C.J. 1980. Monoclonal antibodies which recognize different cell types in the rat retina. *Nature* **286**:231.

Eisenbarth, G.S., F.S. Walsh, and M. Nirenberg. 1979. Monoclonal antibody to a plasma membrane antigen of neurons. *Proc. Natl. Acad. Sci.* **76**:4913.

Galfre, G., S.C. Howe, C. Milstein, G.W. Butcher, and J.C. Howard. 1977. Antibodies to major histocompatibility antigens produced by hybrid cell lines. *Nature* **266:**550.

Goldschneider, I. and A.A. Moscona. 1972. Tissue-specific cell-surface antigens in embryonic cells. *J. Cell Biol.* **53:**435.

Hausman, R.E. and A.A. Moscona. 1979. Immunologic detection of retina cognin on the surface of embryonic cells. *Exp. Cell Res.* **119:**191.

Köhler, G. and C. Milstein. 1975. Continuous cultures of fused cells secreting antibody of predefined specificity. *Nature* **256:**495.

Schneider, M.D. and G.S. Eisenbarth. 1979. Transfer plate radioassay using cell monolayers to detect anti-cell surface antibodies produced by lymphocyte hybridomas. *J. Immunol. Methods* **29:**331.

Silver, J. and R.L. Sidman. 1980. A mechanism for the guidance and topographic patterning of retinal ganglion cell axons. *J. Comp. Neurol.* **189:**101.

Sperry, R.W. 1963. Chemoaffinity in the orderly growth of nerve fiber patterns and connections. *Proc. Natl. Acad. Sci.* **50:**703.

Thiery, J.-P., R. Brackenbury, U. Rutishauser, and G.M. Edelman. 1977. Adhesion among neural cells of the chick embryo. II. Purification and characterization of a cell adhesion molecules from neural retina. *J. Biol. Chem.* **252:**6841.

Trisler, G.D., M.D. Schneider, and M. Nirenberg. 1981. A topographic gradient of molecules in retina can be used to identify neuron position. *Proc. Natl. Acad. Sci.* **78:**2145.

Trisler, G.D., M.A. Donlon, W.G. Shain, and H.G. Coon. 1979. Recognition of antigenic differences among neurons using antiserums to clonal neural retina hybrid cells. *Fed. Proc.* **38:**2368.

Monoclonal Antibodies to the Frog Nerve-Muscle Synapse

STEVEN BURDEN

Department of Anatomy
Harvard Medical School
Boston, Massachusetts 02115

• More is known about the neuromuscular synapse than any other synapse in the body. Its relative simplicity and accessibility have provided us with a fairly detailed account of what a synapse looks like and how a synapse functions. We remain, however, rather poorly informed about the biochemical events involved in the formation of this highly specialized region of cell-to-cell contact.

Two macromolecules are known to be highly concentrated at neuromuscular synapses: the acetylcholine receptor (AChR) and acetylcholinesterase. It is clear that nerve and muscle must interact during development in order to organize these macromolecules at the synapse (Anderson and Cohen 1977; Frank and Fischbach 1979; Rubin et al. 1979). At present, however, we have little insight into the mechanisms involved in this nerve-muscle interaction and the ensuing differentiation of the synapse. One hindrance to a detailed examination of the sequence of steps in synapse formation is our rather limited knowledge of the macromolecules present at synapses; AChR and acetylcholinesterase are the only such macromolecules that have been characterized as of now. To gain further insight into the mechanisms involved in the formation of synapses, we have begun to produce monoclonal antibodies that are directed against components of the neuromuscular synapse.

STRUCTURE OF THE NEUROMUSCULAR JUNCTION

• The cellular components of the neuromuscular junction are the nerve, muscle, and Schwann cells (Fig. 1). Frog cutaneous pectoris

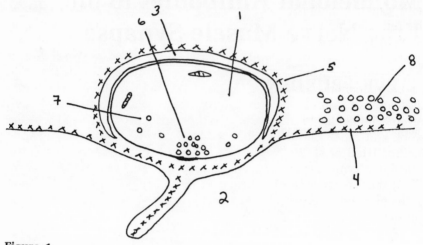

Figure 1

Schematic diagram of the frog neuromuscular synapse as seen by electron microscopy in cross section. Structures described in the text and illustrated here include the nerve terminal (1), myofiber (2), Schwann cell (3), myofiber basal lamina (4), Schwann cell basal lamina (5), active zones (6), synaptic vesicles (7), and reticular lamina (8).

muscle contains about 500 muscle fibers, innervated by approximately 25 motor neurons. The nerve terminal of the synapse lies in a shallow groove of the muscle fiber and is covered by the Schwann cell (Fig. 1). Both nerve and muscle contain specialized subcellular structures at the synaptic site. For the nerve terminal, this includes the collection of vesicles that store and release acetylcholine as well as macromolecular structures of the presynaptic membrane that regulate transmitter release. The postsynaptic muscle membrane has a dense filamentous network, analogous to the postsynaptic density at nerve-nerve synapses. The muscle membrane at the synapse is highly invaginated, and these membrane folds are termed junctional folds; acetylcholine receptors are restricted to the crests and upper sides of these junctional folds, and the filamentous postsynaptic network is also concentrated in this region.

An extracellular matrix component of largely unknown composition encircles the muscle fiber and caps the Schwann cell. This extracellular matrix, known as basal lamina, also penetrates the synaptic cleft and into the junctional folds. The basal lamina is a layer of extracellular material that is approximately 250 Å thick in muscle; hence, basal lamina is an electron microscopy term. In the light microscope, it is a component of a larger structure called the basement membrane, which is composed of basal lamina in combination with a matrix of fibrillar collagen and glycosaminoglycans known as the reticular lamina. The basal lamina contains nonfibrillar collagen of types IV and V (Carlson et al. 1973; Burgeson et al. 1976), uncharacterized glycosaminoglycans, and perhaps other macromolecules. It is known to contain the enzyme acetylcholinesterase (McMahan et al. 1978); histochemical staining for this enzyme in whole tissue demonstrates localization of reaction product to the synaptic cleft. Although several molecular forms of the enzyme exist in muscle tissue, in the chick and rat the fastest sedimentating form is localized to synaptic regions (Hall et al. 1973; Vigry et al. 1976). Furthermore, in electric fish the enzyme has an elongated tail (Dudai et al. 1973; Rieger et al. 1973) that is sensitive to collagenase (Johnson et al. 1977); this form of the enzyme is localized to the synaptic region of the myofiber basal lamina.

AChR is localized to the synaptic site, embedded in the muscle membrane overlying the postsynaptic density. Suitably conjugated derivatives of α-bungarotoxin have been used to observe the distribution of receptors by light and electron microscopy. In normal muscle, acetylcholinesterase staining and α-bungarotoxin binding are coincident at the synapse. Acetylcholinesterase marks the synaptic regions of the extracellular matrix, whereas α-bungarotoxin marks the synaptic region of the muscle membrane. Comparison of the relative positions of the two markers under conditions in which the junctional structure has been perturbed, such as during regeneration following injury to nerve or muscle, provides evidence for interaction of the extracellular matrix with cellular components during synaptogenesis.

MORPHOGENESIS OF THE NEUROMUSCULAR JUNCTION

• Morphogenesis of the neuromuscular junction has been studied under two situations: normal development and regeneration. In normal development, both nerve and muscle interact to form a synapse. Experimentally this site is defined as the site of accumulation of AChRs (Anderson and Cohen 1977; Frank and Fischbach 1979). Prior to synapse formation, receptors are uniformly distributed along the muscle fiber. After the motor nerve has contacted the muscle fiber, receptors accumulate at the synapse. After some time, the number of extrajunctional receptors decreases. In the adult, the density of receptors is 5000-fold greater at synaptic sites than in extrajunctional regions (Fambrough and Hartzell 1972; Fertuck and Salpeter 1976).

Following denervation, receptors remain concentrated at the original synaptic site, but new receptors appear over the entire muscle cell surface. This is the origin of the phenomenon of denervation sensitivity, in which sensitivity to iontophoretically applied acetylcholine spreads along the muscle fiber, which prior to denervation was localized at synaptic sites. After nerve regeneration, receptors once more become restricted to the point of nerve-muscle contact.

ROLE OF THE EXTRACELLULAR MATRIX IN REGENERATION OF THE NEUROMUSCULAR JUNCTION

• Reformation of the neuromuscular junction can occur successfully after destruction of both nerve and muscle. After damage to nerve and muscle, both nerve terminals and muscle fibers degenerate and are phagocytized, but the muscle fiber's basal lamina sheath remains intact (Carlson 1972; Vracko and Benditt 1972). Even in the absence of nerve and muscle, structures remain at the original synaptic site, which allows one to identify where the synapse was (Sanes et al. 1978; Burden et al. 1979). These include the Schwann cell, the projection of the basal lamina that previously penetrated the postsynaptic folds, and the enzyme acetylcholinesterase. After some time, axons regenerate to the muscle and new myofibers form within the original myofiber's basal lamina from the proliferation and fusion of mononucleated satellite cells. These regenerated axons form synapses with the regenerated myofibers precisely at the original synaptic site (Sanes et al. 1979). If axons are allowed to regenerate to the muscle, but muscle regeneration is prevented, axons unerringly return to the original synaptic site on the basal lamina, and active zones form precisely across from the projections of basal lamina that previously penetrated the folds of the postsynaptic membrane (Sanes et al. 1979). Thus, the presence of the muscle cell is not necessary for either precise reinnervation of original synaptic sites or for the morphological differentiation of these regenerated nerve terminals. Moreover, if axon regeneration is prevented but myofibers are allowed to regenerate, AChRs accumulate and membrane folds form precisely at the original synaptic site on the basal lamina (Burden et al. 1979). Furthermore, if muscle fibers are allowed to regenerate in the absence of both nerve and Schwann cells, receptors accumulate and folds develop specifically at the original synaptic site (S.J. Burden, in prep.). Thus, in the absence of nerve, muscle, and Schwann cells, information remains at the original synaptic site that is instructive for the differentiation of both regenerated nerve terminals and a highly specialized postsynaptic membrane. The most prominent extracellular structure that remains at the neuromuscular synapse after removal of all cells is the synaptic portion of the myofiber's basal lamina. Therefore, the synaptic portion of the myofiber basal lamina, or a structure closely associated with the basal lamina, contains and stores information for the differentiation of both regenerating nerve and muscle.

At present, we have little information concerning the molecular composition of the synaptic basal lamina and little insight into how the basal lamina can trigger the differentiation of regenerating nerve and muscle. To study synaptic development in greater detail, we have begun to define and characterize macromolecular components of neuromuscular synapses by using monoclonal antibodies.

GENERATION OF MONOCLONAL ANTIBODIES TO THE EXTRACELLULAR MATRIX OF THE FROG NEUROMUSCULAR JUNCTION

• The immunogen consisted of material isolated from *Torpedo californica* electric organ on the basis of its insolubility in nonionic detergents and in high and low salt concentrations (Cohen et al. 1972; Carlson et al. 1973; Duguid and Rafferty 1973; Burgeson et al. 1976). Spleen cells of immunized mice were fused with the myeloma parent NS1 (Oi and Herzenberg 1980). Approximately 5×10^5 large, viable cells were plated per culture in 24-cluster Linbro wells. Supernatants from these cultures were screened using indirect immunofluorescence on fresh-frozen sections of frog muscle. Cells from interesting wells were cloned by limited-dilution plating on feeder layers of peritoneal cells. Only those cultures whose supernatants stained at synaptic sites, as identified by tetramethyl-rhodamine (TMR)-conjugated α-bungarotoxin, or that had other interesting staining distributions were cloned. The supernatant staining was visualized using fluorescein-conjugated goat anti−mouse IgG (Fig. 2). This screening procedure retrieved clones useful for histological studies.

CHARACTERISTICS OF MONOCLONAL ANTIBODIES STAINING FROG NEUROMUSCULAR JUNCTION

Monoclonal antibody number 1

• This antibody stains intensely at the synaptic region of normal frog muscle. It does not cross-react with rat or mouse. After denervation, staining appears around the periphery of the muscle fiber, although a higher intensity is retained at the synaptic site (Fig. 3). The antigen disappears after removal of both nerve and muscle. Staining with this antibody is not blocked by α-bungarotoxin, nor does the antibody bind to affinity-purified AChRs. The binding test was performed by measuring the amount of radioactivity sedimented after addition of Staph A to radioiodinated bungarotoxin-receptor complexes incubated with the monoclonal antibody. Furthermore, the staining is insen-

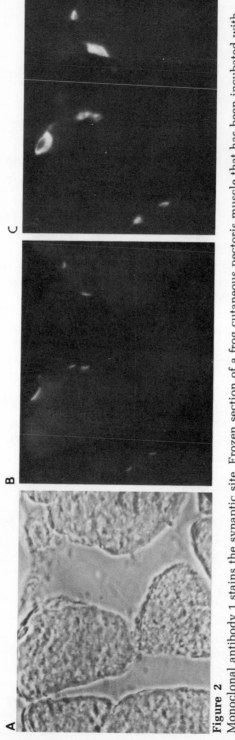

Figure 2

Monoclonal antibody 1 stains the synaptic site. Frozen section of a frog cutaneous pectoris muscle that has been incubated with TMR−α-bungarotoxin and monoclonal antibody 1 followed by goat anti−mouse IgG coupled to fluorescein. (A) Phase optics; (B) rhodamine optics demonstrating synaptic sites; (C) fluorescein optics illustrating antibody binding.

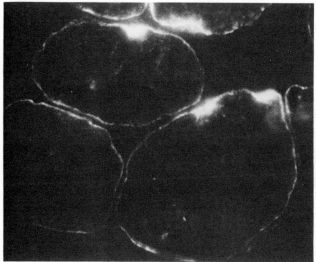

Figure 3
Monoclonal antibody 1 stains the synaptic site and extra-synaptic areas following denervation. Frozen section of a frog cutaneous pectoris muscle that had been denervated for six days. The section was incubated with antibodies and toxin as described in the legend to Fig. 2; only the antibody binding is illustrated here. Bright staining persists at the synaptic site, but staining is now also present at extrasynaptic regions.

sitive to pretreatment of the sections with collagenase, indicating that the antigen is probably not structurally associated with collagen. It is now clear that the antigen is localized intracellularly: Staining is not observed in whole muscle but only in muscle that has been fixed and permeabilized with Triton X-100.

Biochemical characterization of the antigens reacting with antibody 1 has begun. *T. californica* proteins analyzed on SDS-polyacrylamide gel electrophoresis and transferred to paper have been stained with the antibody. No proteins solubilized by low-ionic-strength buffer or 2% Triton X-100 are labeled by the antibody. However, several Coomassie-blue-stained bands in a high-ionic-strength soluble fraction react with the antibody.

Monoclonal antibody number 2

This antibody also stains frog, but not rat or mouse, neuromuscular junctions. In addition, there is staining at the muscle fiber periphery.

Blood vessels and nerve terminals are also stained. Pretreatment with collagenase abolishes the staining, suggesting that the antibody recognizes an antigen associated with the extracellular matrix.

Monoclonal antibody number 3

This antibody stains near synaptic sites but in a somewhat different pattern than α-bungarotoxin. It appears to cap the nerve terminal and to extend laterally beyond the synaptic site. The staining appears to be excluded from the synaptic cleft and is often thicker at the edges of the synapse. Antibody staining at the synaptic site persists after denervation. Staining is also present within intramuscular nerve trunks and persists there after denervation.

To ask whether this antibody stained nerve-nerve cholinergic synapses as well as the neuromuscular junction, the frog cardiac ganglion was stained with horseradish-peroxidase-coupled second antibody following incubation with monoclonal antibody 3. In this preparation the principal neurons of the ganglion are known to receive most of their synaptic input from boutons clustered over their axon hillocks. Preliminary results suggest that there is reaction product localized to synaptic sites.

INTERMEDIATE FILAMENTS AT THE NEUROMUSCULAR JUNCTION

• Two facts together suggest that intermediate filaments are important components of the nerve-muscle synapse. Electron microscope studies of preparations stained with peroxidase-coupled α-bungarotoxin show that the filamentous network of the postsynaptic density closely follows the distribution of AChRs on the upper portion, but not along the bottom, of the junctional folds. High-voltage electron microscope studies (Ellisman et al. 1976) showed that this postsynaptic web is in part composed of intermediate filaments.

STAINING PATTERNS OF MONOCLONAL ANTIBODIES TO INTERMEDIATE FILAMENTS IN SKELETAL MUSCLE

• Two monoclonal antibodies of different specificities have been used to observe intermediate filaments at the frog neuromuscular junction. The first interacts with all known types of intermediate filaments (see Pruss et al., this volume). In addition to staining with high intensity at frog muscle synaptic sites, this antibody also stained within the muscle fiber cytoplasm. This intracellular staining may be attributable to the presence of the intermediate filament proteins desmin and vimentin. The synaptic staining is due to an as yet unidentified antigen that presumably shares a determinant common to other intermediate filament proteins.

The second antibody used is specific for tonofilaments (a gift from E.B. Lane, Imperial Cancer Research Fund, London; antibody to mammalian tonofilaments, PtK2 cell line), the intermediate filament type that is characteristic of epithelial cells. This antibody brightly stained frog muscle synapses but not within muscle fiber cytoplasm nor within nerve or Schwann cells. Following denervation, however, staining persisted at the synapse but also appeared, at lower intensity, in extrajunctional regions. Like monoclonal antibody 1, the anti-tonofilament antibody was not blocked by α-bungarotoxin, nor did it bind AChRs, implying that it does not recognize a shared determinant of tonofilaments and AChRs. The redistribution of staining of monoclonal antibody 1 and of the anti-tonofilament antibody following denervation is suggestive of a role in synapse formation or stabilization. Furthermore, staining is observed in whole muscle only after Triton treatment, demonstrating that the antigen is an intracellular synaptic macromolecule.

SUMMARY

• Monoclonal antibodies with specific binding to the frog neuromuscular junction have been prepared using insoluble matrix material of T. *californica* electric organ as an immunogen. Three of the many that were isolated were described in this paper. The first stains only at the synapse in normal muscle but spreads around the muscle periphery following denervation. The recognized antigen is not the AChR. The second stains at the synapse and along the muscle fiber periphery as well as around blood vessels and the nerve terminal. Its sensitivity to collagenase suggests it is an extracellular matrix component. The third antibody stains both nerve-nerve and nerve-muscle synapses.

The presence of intermediate filaments at the frog neuromuscular junction was also explored using monoclonal antibodies. A monoclonal antibody that reacts with all known intermediate filament types stains with high intensity at the synaptic site. A monoclonal antibody directed specifically against mammalian tonofilaments stained precisely and specifically at normal frog synapses and stained around the muscle fiber periphery, as well, following denervation.

This work shows that the generation of monoclonal antibodies to the frog neuromuscular junction is a viable approach for analysis of its structure. The discovery of antigens other than the AChR that appear at extrajunctional sites following denervation opens new territory for inquiry into how the synapse is established and maintained.

REFERENCES

Anderson, M.J. and M.W. Cohen. 1977. Nerve-induced and spontaneous redistribution of acetylcholine receptors on cultured muscle cells. *J. Physiol.* **268:**757.

Burden, S.J., P.B. Sargent, and U.J. McMahan. 1979. Acetylcholine receptors in regenerating muscle accumulate at original synaptic sites in the absence of nerve. *J. Cell Biol.* **82:**412.

Burgeson, R.E., F.A. Adeli, I.I. Kaitila, and D.W. Hollister. 1976. Foetal membrane collagens: Identification of two new collagen alpha chains. *Proc. Natl. Acad. Sci.* **3:**2579.

Carlson, B.M. 1972. The regeneration of skeletal muscle—A review. *Am. J. Anat.* **137:**119.

Carlson, E.C., K. Brendel, J.T. Hjelle, and E. Meezan. 1973. Ultrastructural and biochemical analysis of isolated basement membranes from kidney glomeruli and tubules and brain and retinal micro-vessels. *J. Ultrastruct. Res.* **62:**26.

Cohen, J.B., M. Weber, M. Huschet, and J.-P. Changeux. 1972. Purification from *Torpedo marmorata* electric tissue membrane fragments particularly rich in cholinergic receptor protein. *FEBS Lett.* **26:**43.

Dudai, Y., M. Herzberg, and I. Silman. 1973. Molecular structures of acetylcholinesterase from electric organ tissue of the electric eel. *Proc. Natl. Acad. Sci.* **70:**2473.

Duguid, J.R. and M.A. Rafferty. 1973. Fractionation and partial characterization of membrane particles from *Torpedo californica* electroplax. *Biochemistry* **12:**3593.

Ellisman, M.A., J.E. Rash, A. Staehlin, and K.R. Porter. 1976. Studies of excitable membranes. *J. Cell Biol.* **68:**752.

Fambrough, D. and H.C. Hartzell. 1972. Acetylcholine receptors: Number and distribution at neuromuscular junctions in rat diaphragm. *Science* **176:**189.

Fertuck, H.C. and M.M. Salpeter. 1976. Quantitation of junctional and extrajunctional acetylcholine receptors by electron microscope autoradiography after ^{125}I-α-bungarotoxin binding at mouse neuromuscular junctions. *J. Cell Biol.* **69:**144.

Frank, E. and G.D. Fischbach. 1979. Early events in neuromuscular junction formation *in vitro*. *J. Cell Biol.* **83:**143.

Hall, Z.W. 1973. Multiple forms of acetylcholinesterase and their distribution in endplate and non-endplate regions of rat diaphragm muscle. *J. Neurobiol.* **4:**343.

Johnson, C.D., S.P. Smith, and R.L. Russell. 1977. *Electrophorus electricus* acetylcholinesterases; separation and selective modification by collagenase. *J. Neurochem.* **28:**617.

McMahan, U.J., J.R. Sanes, and L.M. Marshall. 1978. Cholinesterase is associated with the basal lamina at the neuromuscular junction. *Nature* **271:**172.

Oi, V. and L.A. Herzenberg. 1980. Immunoglobulin-producing hybrid cell lines. In *Selected methods in cellular immunology* (ed. B.B. Mishell and S.M. Shugi), vol. 3, p. 51. Freeman, San Francisco.

Rieger, F., S. Bon, and J. Massoulié. 1973. Observation par microscopie électronique des formes allongées et globulaires de l'acetylcholinestérase de gymmote (*Electrophorus electricus*). *Eur. J. Biochem.* **34**:539.

Rubin, L.L., S.M. Schurtze, and G.D. Fischbach. 1979. Accumulation of acetylcholinesterase at newly formed nerve-muscle synapses. *Dev. Biol.* **69**:46.

Sanes, J.R., L.M. Marshall, and U.J. McMahan. 1978. Reinnervation of muscle fiber basal lamina after removal of muscle fibers. *J. Cell Biol.* **78**:176.

Vigny, M., L. DiGiamberardino, J.Y. Couraud, F. Rieger, and J. Koenig. 1976. Molecular forms of chicken acetylcholinesterase: Effect of denervation. *FEBS Lett.* **69**:277.

Vracko, R. and E.P. Benditt. 1972. Basal lamina: The scaffold for orderly cell replacement. *J. Cell Biol.* **55**:406.

Monoclonal Antibodies to Extracellular Matrix Antigens in Chicken Skeletal Muscle

ELLEN K. BAYNE, JOHN GARDNER, and DOUGLAS M. FAMBROUGH

Department of Embryology
Carnegie Institution of Washington
Baltimore, Maryland 21210

• The importance of extracellular matrix during myogenesis and synaptogenesis is becoming increasingly evident. Not only does extracellular matrix serve as a scaffold for maintenance of tissue structure and a substratum for attachment and migration of cells during embryonic development and tissue regeneration, but extracellular matrix also appears to exert a directive influence on synapse organization. Specializations within the basal lamina at frog neuromuscular junctions are now thought to induce both synaptic differentiation of regenerating nerve terminals (Burden et al. 1979) and accumulation of acetylcholine receptors within the "postsynaptic" membrane of regenerating muscle (Sanes et al. 1978). Furthermore, through use of immunohistochemical techniques, molecular differences between synaptic and extrasynaptic regions of basal lamina have been demonstrated (Sanes and Hall 1979).

Clearly, extracellular matrix is both complex and highly ordered. Skeletal muscle extracellular matrix has not been well characterized, however, and its cellular sources remain largely a matter for speculation. We have generated a set of monoclonal antibodies that allow us to identify extracellular matrix antigens in vivo and in vitro. These antibodies have been developed for use in cultures of embryonic chicken muscle. Tissue culture is convenient for biochemical analysis, and cultures are easily manipulatable in experiments that attempt to identify antigen function. Any promising in vitro results can be compared to in vivo studies to confirm their generality. Three important aims of this work are: (1) to determine the composition of chicken skeletal muscle extracellular matrix; (2) to determine which cells synthesize individual components and how these components are assembled into the matrix; and (3) to determine the functions of the extracellular matrix during muscle development and at maturity.

In this paper we first describe our procedures for generating monoclonal antibodies and illustrate some representative staining patterns of different antibodies on frozen tissue sections and in muscle cultures. We then discuss an antibody (designated number 6) that has proven to be very useful in making pure myotube cultures and describe some preliminary analysis of extracellular matrix components in these cultures. Finally, our observations utilizing an antibody (number 33) that is targeted against an extracellular matrix antigen that codistributes with acetylcholine receptors are discussed.

GENERATION OF MONOCLONAL ANTIBODIES

• The immunogen was prepared by washing a homogenate of embryonic day-14 chick leg muscle with phosphate-buffered saline (PBS) to remove soluble proteins. After emulsification with complete Freund's adjuvant, the preparation was injected intraperitoneally into BALB/c mice. Animals were boosted one month after the initial injection. Three days later, spleen cells were fused with cells of the nonsecreting myeloma line SP2/0, according to the protocol of Kennett et al. (1979), using polyethylene glycol 1000 as a fusagen. Hybridomas were selected by their ability to grow in hypoxanthine, aminopterin, thymidine (HAT) medium. A monoclonal antibody to fibronectin was also prepared by the same method. In this case the immunogen consisted of fibronectin extracted from tertiary chick fibroblast cultures with 1 M urea (Yamada et al. 1975, 1976) and further purified by affinity chromatography on a collagen-agarose column (Engvell and Ruoslahti 1977).

The screening procedure was designed to retrieve clones producing antibodies that would be useful in morphological and biochemical studies of muscle cultures. Hybridoma antibodies were screened in two ways: (1) use of an iodinated second antibody, directed against mouse Fab fragments, to monitor binding of monoclonal antibodies to unfixed chick muscle cultures; and (2) indirect immunofluorescent staining of cultured muscle and of frozen tissue slices.

Interesting hybrids were cloned in soft agar from one to three times. Prior to the harvesting of individual clones, the cultures were covered with a layer of agar that contained anti-isotype antibody. Formation of precipitin rings around clones allowed identification of antibody type and selection of high secretors. Cloned hybrids were grown as ascites tumors in mice. Immunoglobulin was purified from ascites fluid by ammonium sulfate precipitation, followed by gel filtration on Pharmacia Ultragel ACA22 and/or ion exchange chromatography on DEAE-cellulose. Each antibody has been obtained in 150–200-mg quantities. Standardized amounts of antibodies were used in experiments.

Immunofluorescence Staining Patterns

• Out of 35 clones retrieved by the screening procedure, about 17 appeared to stain extracellular matrix of frozen muscle slices and unfixed muscle cultures. The staining patterns of these 17 antibodies have been classified into seven distinct groups. It is not yet known whether those antibodies with similar distribution of binding recognize the same antigen or different but closely associated antigens. Differences among the seven patterns include distance of staining from the sarcolemma, uniformity of distribution, and substructure, such as patchiness or weblike forms. Four of these patterns in tissue slices are illustrated in Figure 1. The muscle we utilized for staining had been treated with tetramethyl-rhodamine-labeled α-bungarotoxin

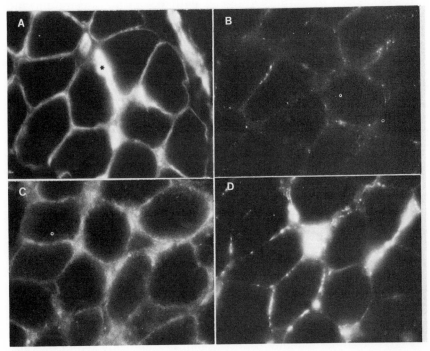

Figure 1
Immunofluorescent staining of chicken skeletal muscle cross sections with monoclonal antibodies to different components of the extracellular matrix. (A) Continuous rings of stain encircling the muscle fibers in close apposition. This antibody, 33, also stains blood vessels. The asterisk marks the site of a concentration of both antibody 33 and tetramethyl-rhodamine-conjugated α-bungarotoxin binding. (B) Punctate accumulations of antigen 3 between muscle fibers. (C) Staining of the extracellular matrix with antibody 15. A diffuse, weblike fluorescence extends through the endomysium. (D) Staining of fibronectin with hybridoma B3 antibody.

prior to sectioning. α-Bungarotoxin binds specifically and virtually irreversibly to acetylcholine receptors within skeletal muscle and allows identification of the receptor-rich endplate regions. When the sectioned muscle is then stained with monoclonal antibody and a fluorescein-isothiocyanate-conjugated second antibody, the spatial relationships of particular antigens to neuromuscular junctions can be assessed. The region marked by an asterisk in Figure 1A was identified as a motor endplate. Intense staining of this region is obtained utilizing antibody 33. In contrast, the other antibodies illustrated in Figure 1 apparently do not extend into synaptic clefts. Fibronectin staining (Fig. 1D), for example, was never observed to colocalize with acetylcholine receptors.

Striking differences in antigen distribution are also observed in muscle cultures. Immunofluorescent staining demonstrates differential association of various antigens with cells and substratum and elaboration of different antigens into morphologically distinguishable networks. Some of the staining patterns we observed are illustrated in Figure 2. The inhomogeneous distribution of matrix antigens in culture suggests that an in vitro equivalent of the extracellular matrix of intact muscle is formed.

SECRETION OF MATRIX COMPONENTS BY MUSCLE CELLS

• A question that interests us is the role of various cell types during matrix biogenesis. To address this problem, it becomes necessary to prepare cultures containing pure cell populations. One of the monoclonal antibodies that we have (antibody 6) has been successfully utilized for this purpose. This antibody recognizes a membrane component present on myoblasts and fibroblasts but not mature myotubes. When added to cultures, together with guinea pig complement, it causes complement-mediated lysis of target cells, leaving cultures consisting of almost pure myotubes. A treated culture is illustrated in Figure 3. More than 97% of the nuclei are in multinucleated myotubes, and many of the remaining nuclei are in mononucleated, differentiated muscle cells.

To determine whether differentiated muscle cells synthesize matrix components, we incubated these pure myotube cultures with radioactive amino acids and analyzed secreted products on SDS-polyacrylamide gels (Fig. 4). Cultures incubated with [^{35}S]methionine secrete a complex array of radioactively labeled polypeptides ranging in size from >300,000 to <40,000 daltons. Certain bands can incorporate large amounts of [^{3}H]proline and are collagenase-sensitive, suggesting that they are collagens. Also among the secreted components is fibronectin, which appears as a doublet with an apparent molecular weight of ~ 230,000. These bands are selectively precipitated by our

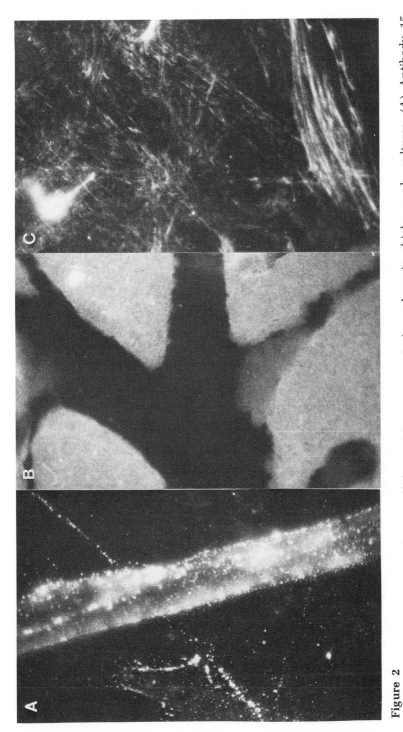

Figure 2
Immunofluorescent staining of extracellular matrix components in embryonic chick. muscle cultures. (A) Antibody 15 preferentially stains cells in the culture, although some staining of the substratum is seen. (B) Antibody 9 produces a diffuse staining of the culture substratum. (C) Anti-fibronectin antibody, B3, stains structurally complex networks associated with both cells and substratum.

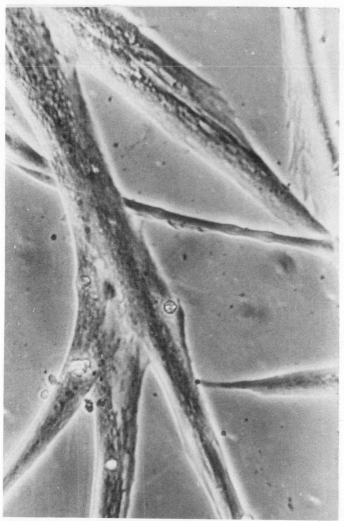

Figure 3
Phase micrograph of a pure myotube culture prepared by treatment with antibody 6 plus complement. To achieve the elimi-
nation of mononucleated cells, 1 μg of hybridoma 6 IgM per
ml and 5% guinea pig complement were used in complete
medium for 1 hr at 37°C.

anti-fibronectin antibody. By immunofluorescent staining, all of the
matrix antigens detected in conventional muscle cultures and in
sectioned muscle have been observed in pure myotube cultures prepared using antibody 6 plus complement. Evidently, muscle cells are
active secretory cells that are capable of synthesizing many compo-

nents of their own matrix. Monoclonal antibodies will be used to analyze further the relationship between the soluble proteins secreted by the myotubes and those of their insoluble matrix.

AN ANTIGEN THAT CODISTRIBUTES WITH ACETYLCHOLINE RECEPTORS

• One antigen (recognized by an antibody designated number 33) has been of particular interest to us because its accumulation on muscle bears a direct relationship to a known membrane constituent, the

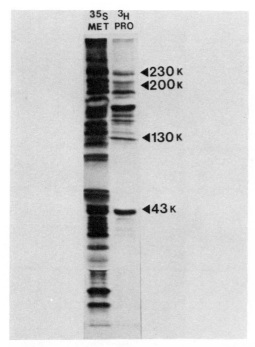

Figure 4
Autoradiograph of a polyacrylamide gel separating secretory products from pure myotube cultures that were metabolically labeled with either [³⁵S]methionine or [³H]proline. The proline-rich components include a fibronectin doublet with an apparent molecular weight of ~ 230,000 and several collagenous peptides in the molecular-weight range of 150,000–200,000. Some approximate molecular weights, based on the electrophoretic migration of standards, are indicated at the right.

acetylcholine receptor. The staining pattern of antibody 33 in a muscle cross section is shown in Figure 1A. The endplate region within the section (identified with an asterisk) stains intensely. Figure 5 perhaps better illustrates the correspondence between antigen 33 and acetylcholine receptors. An endplate stained with tetramethyl-rhodamine-labeled α-bungarotoxin is illustrated in panel B. Panel A shows the same section stained with fluorescein-conjugated antibody. Antigen extends over the entire surface of the muscle. At the neuromuscular junction, concentrations of antigen closely correspond to acetylcholine receptor distribution.

In culture, both myoblasts and myotubes are stained by antibody 33. On myotubes the staining appears as a fine web extending over the cell surface and as dense patches exhibiting intricate substructure. When cultures are treated first with tetramethyl-rhodamine-labeled α-bungarotoxin and then processed for indirect immuno-

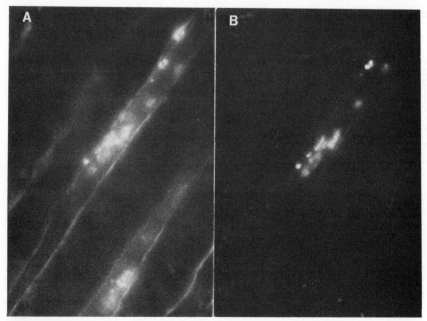

Figure 5
Grazing longitudinal section of chicken anterior latissimus dorsi muscle stained with tetramethyl-rhodamine-conjugated α-bungarotoxin and antibody 33 tagged with fluorescent second antibody. Muscle was first exposed to rhodamine-labeled α-bungarotoxin, then frozen and sectioned longitudinally. Sections were treated with monoclonal antibody 33 and fluorescein-conjugated goat anti−mouse IgG. (A) Fluorescein fluorescence showing the high concentration of antigen 33 at a neuromuscular junction as well as labeling along the muscle surface. (B) Binding of rhodamine-labeled α-bungarotoxin to the same neuromuscular junction.

fluorescence, a codistribution of antigen patches and acetylcholine receptors is evident. An example of this codistribution of antigen 33 and acetylcholine receptors on a cultured myotube is shown in Figure 6. All receptor clusters were coincident with antigen patches, although not all patches of antigen were associated with receptor clusters. The observation that antigen accumulates on cells prior to the formation of receptor clusters and that all receptor clusters have associated antigen raises the possibility that antigen 33 may play a role in the organization of receptors within muscle membranes.

The pattern of accumulation of antigen 33 on the surfaces of myotubes appeared identical in fibroblast-containing as well as fibroblast-free muscle cultures (obtained by preplating cell suspensions and later killing any fibroblasts growing in culture with antibody 6 and complement). This accumulation of antigen on muscle surfaces does not appear to depend on the presence of fibroblasts within the cultures. Fibroblasts do, however, appear capable of secreting antigen 33. In fibroblast cultures, accumulation of antigen 33 shows a cell-density dependence. Although only a small amount of antigen 33 is detected by immunofluorescence in subconfluent cultures, once fibroblasts reach confluence they elaborate a complex antigen matrix that extends over the cell monolayer (Fig. 7). Clearly then, antigen 33 is not muscle-specific. The relation of the antigen to myotube and fibroblast surfaces, however, seems to be quite different.

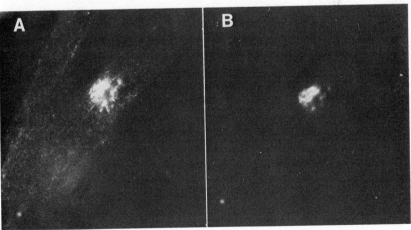

Figure 6
Colocalization of antigen 33 and acetylcholine receptors on a chick myotube in culture. The unfixed culture was exposed to tetramethyl-rhodamine-labeled α-bungarotoxin, then to antibody 33, and finally to a fluorescein-labeled goat anti–mouse IgG. (A) Fluorescein fluorescence of an antigen-33 patch on a myotube cell surface. (B) Rhodamine fluorescence showing clustered acetylcholine receptors to which α-bungarotoxin had bound.

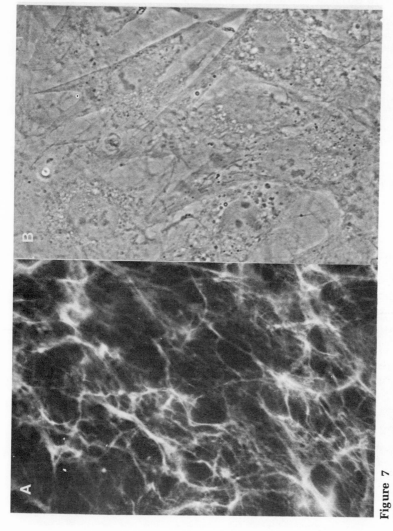

Figure 7

Fluorescent staining of antigen 33 in a confluent embryonic chick fibroblast culture. The unfixed culture was exposed first to antibody 33 and then to a fluorescein-conjugated goat anti–mouse IgG. (A) Fluorescein fluorescence of antigen-33 matrix. (B) Phase micrograph of the same culture.

BIOCHEMICAL CHARACTERIZATION OF ANTIGEN 33

• Partial purification of antigen 33 from late chick embryo skeletal muscle has been achieved by a procedure involving homogenization and washes in high salt concentration followed by extraction with 0.5 M NaCl at neutral pH. Major collagens were removed from extracts by fractional salt precipitation (Timpl et al. 1979). When such a preparation is run on a sucrose gradient, the antigen sediments as a broad peak at 16–18S. This peak separates from the sedimentation profiles of two other extracellular matrix antigens followed in the same preparation. The antigen does not appear to be sensitive to treatment with purified collagenase and is not removed from solution by differential salt precipitation. It is thus not likely to be one of the major collagens. The antigen may also be distinct from laminin, a basement membrane glycoprotein that has been isolated from a mouse tumor. In solutions containing low-ionic-strength urea, antigen 33 is absorbed to DEAE-cellulose, unlike laminin, which remains unbound during anion exchange chromatography. It may turn out that antigen 33 is a novel matrix molecule.

SUMMARY

• Components of the basal lamina, which ensheaths skeletal muscle fibers and extends through the synaptic clefts at neuromuscular junctions, appear to play important roles in synapse organization. Monoclonal antibodies provide a powerful approach for identification and analysis of extracellular matrix constituents. One antibody that we have produced, antibody 6, has proven useful in making pure myotube cultures for studying the secretory and matrix components synthesized by these cells in the absence of fibroblasts. Another antibody, 33, binds a basal lamina antigen that codistributes with acetylcholine receptors. In culture, patches of this antigen are associated with all receptor clusters. The appearance of antigen 33 precedes that of acetylcholine receptor clusters. The possibility that this extracellular antigen plays a role in acetylcholine receptor localization is currently under investigation.

ACKNOWLEDGMENTS

• This research has been supported in part by a grant from the Muscular Dystrophy Association and in part by grant NS 16542 from the National Institute of Neurological and Communicative Disorders and Stroke, National Institutes of Health.

REFERENCES

Burden, S.J., P.B. Sargent, and U.J. McMahan. 1979. Acetylcholine receptors in regenerating muscle accumulate at the original synaptic sites in the absence of the nerve. *J. Cell Biol.* **82:**412.

Engvell, E. and E. Ruoslahti. 1977. Binding of a soluble form of fibroblast surface protein, fibronectin, to collagen. *Int. J. Cancer* **20:**1.

Kennett, R.H., K.A. Denis, A.S. Tong, and N.R. Klinman. 1978. Hybrid plasmacytoma production: Fusions with adult spleen cells, monoclonal spleen fragments, neonatal spleen cells and human spleen cells. *Curr. Top. Microbiol. Immunol.* **81:**77.

Sanes, J.R. and Z.W. Hall. 1979. Antibodies that bind specifically to synaptic sites on muscle fiber basal lamina. *J. Cell Biol.* **83:**357.

Sanes, J.R., L.M. Marshall, and U.J. McMahan. 1978. Reinnervation of muscle fiber basal lamina after removal of myofibers. *J. Cell Biol.* **78:**176.

Timpl, R., H. Rohde, P.G. Robey, S.I. Rennard, J.M. Foidart, and G.R. Martin. 1979. Laminin—A glycoprotein from basement membranes. *J. Biol. Chem.* **254:**9933.

Yamada, K.M., S.S. Yamada, and I. Pastan. 1975. The major cell surface glycoprotein of chick embryo fibroblasts is an agglutinin. *Proc. Natl. Acad. Sci.* **72:**3158.

————. 1976. Cell surface protein partially restores morphology, adhesiveness, and contact inhibition of movement to transformed fibroblasts. *Proc. Natl. Acad. Sci.* **73:**1217.

Effects of Monoclonal Antibodies on the Cell Surface of Cultured Myogenic Cells

JEFFREY M. GREVE and DAVID I. GOTTLIEB

Department of Anatomy and Neurobiology
Washington University School of Medicine
St. Louis, Missouri 63110

• In principle, monoclonal antibodies might be used to dissect the molecular machinery on the cell surface that is responsible for cell-cell recognition. All recent models of cell-cell recognition assume that repertoires of proteins on appropriate cell surfaces interact to insure proper cell-cell recognition (Frazier and Glaser 1979; Gottlieb and Glaser 1980). Some or all of the proteins are likely to be immunogenic, allowing the production of monoclonal antibodies. A subset of these antibodies is probably directed against "active sites" and should therefore block cell recognition. But what if monoclonal antibodies to cell-surface components have nonspecific effects? Antibodies and lectins cause profound changes when they bind to cell-surface antigens, including patching, capping, and global modulation of cell-surface protein mobility (Schlessinger et al. 1977). Perhaps the effects of bound monoclonal antibodies will be so complex as to preclude analysis.

The present experiments were undertaken to throw some light on just what the effects of monoclonal antibodies on living embryonic cells are. Chick embryonic myogenic cells were chosen because they fuse, differentiate, and form synapses in vitro. Each of these steps can be quantified by relatively simple assays. The basic experiment consisted of obtaining monoclonal antibodies that bound to the surfaces of muscle cells and noting the effects of the antibodies on the cultured cells.

GENERATION OF MONOCLONAL ANTIBODIES BINDING TO THE MUSCLE CELL SURFACE

• Material for immunization consisted of primary tissue or cultured cells. Monoclonal antibodies were prepared according to standard methods (Galfre et al. 1977). Active wells were screened by a radioimmunoassay on cultured muscle using a rabbit anti—mouse IgG as secondary antibody. To differentiate binding to the living cell surface from binding to dead cells that contaminate cultures, an autoradiographic visualization method was used. Muscle cultures were treated with hybridoma antibody and iodinated secondary antibody. Disposition of the grains on the autoradiograph indicated which antibodies bound to the majority of cells and hence could be assumed to be binding to living cell surfaces. Fourteen such clones were chosen for study. Large quantities of antibody were prepared by ammonium sulfate fractionation of ascites fluid.

INTERACTION OF MONOCLONAL ANTIBODIES WITH LIVE MUSCLE CELL CULTURES

• Binding of monoclonal antibodies to live cultures of 11-day-old chick thigh muscle was titrated using saturating levels of radioactive second antibody. All 14 antibodies were found to have saturable binding at below 50 μg/ml. To observe effects on myoblast alignment and fusion, 1-day-old cultures were incubated from their second to fourth days in 100–200 μg/ml of antibody. Alterations in morphology, fusion kinetics, and twitching activity were looked for as signs of interference by the antibodies with the normal course of events in culture. Of the 14 antibodies, 12 produced no observable effects.

Even daily additions of these antibodies, which were expected to exceed any capacity of the cells to deplete them from the medium through pinocytosis or other means, had no effect. These results give the important and useful conclusion that saturating occupancy by antibodies of their antigen sites on the muscle cell surface is not an inherently toxic or perturbing situation. This is consistent with results with lymphocytes that continue to function normally when coated with antibodies to a variety of cell-surface antigens. The absence of nonspecific effects due to antibody binding to muscle cells validates the use of monoclonal antibodies as specific probes.

Two antibodies, JG9 and JG22, caused morphological changes. Addition of JG9 to cultures results in formation of very narrow, elongated myotubes. Since these myotubes contained a normal number of nuclei, it does not seem that JG9 lowers the efficiency of fusion. Exposure of cells to JG22 results in large, spherical, refractile structures in which individual nuclei cannot be counted. The morphologies of cultures treated with these two antibodies are shown in Figure 1. The viability of these abnormal cells resulting from exposure to JG9 or JG22 is established because they exclude trypan blue and twitch spontaneously. The reversibility of the effects of exposure to JG9 and

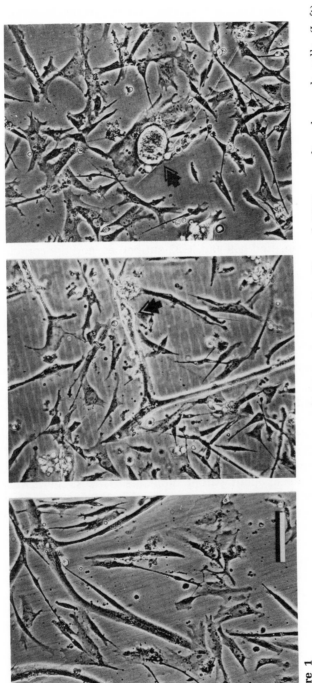

Figure 1

Phase-contrast micrographs showing the effects of monoclonal antibodies JG9 and JG22 on cultured muscle cells. (*Left*) Control cultures grown in the absence of added antibody; (*center*) cells grown for 4 days in the presence of JG9; the arrow points to characteristic swelling of a myotube; (*right*) cells grown for 4 days in the presence of JG22; the arrow points to a large, refractile myogenic cell. Note the normal appearance of fibroblasts. Bar, 100 μm.

the partial reversibility of the effects of JG22 further establish the viability of these cells.

To exclude the possibility that unknown contaminants from the ascites fluid remaining in the antibody preparations were exerting toxic effects, the antibodies were further purified by ion exchange chromatography on a DEAE column, followed by affinity chromatography on a rat anti—mouse-Ig column. These affinity-purified preparations of JG9 and JG22 exerted the same effects as above.

Dose-response studies were done by plotting the percentage of abnormal structures in antibody-treated cultures against the antibody concentration. The amount of antibody producing half-maximal abnormality roughly coincided with that producing half-maximal binding, approximately 3 μg/ml. Somewhat more of JG9 was required than JG22 to produce the same degree of effect.

The lack of effects of the other 12 antibodies, the retention of effect of highly purified JG9 and JG22 antibodies, and the coincidence of the half-maximal points for their binding and dose-response curves strongly support the conclusion that these 2 antibodies exert specific perturbing effects on their targets.

CHARACTERISTICS OF JG9 AND JG22

• Since JG9 and JG22 appeared to have specific effects on muscle cells in culture, these were further characterized. Fab fragments were prepared by mild cysteine reduction and pepsin digestion (J. Greve and D.I. Gottlieb, in prep.). Dose-response studies using the Fab fragments showed that monovalent JG22 retained the full biological effects of the intact antibody. Thus, JG22 can affect cells without cross-linking antigen. In contrast, monovalent JG9 was less than half as effective as its divalent parent molecule. This suggests that the action of JG22 may result directly from blocking of the antigenic determinant by bound antibody, whereas JG9 requires cross-linking to exert its effects. It is also possible that a lower binding affinity for JG9 Fab fragments could also explain these results. Monovalent JG9 would not have sufficient avidity to affect the cultures at the same concentration as divalent JG9, according to this idea.

Since JG9 and JG22 result in different abnormal morphologies when added to muscle cultures, it seemed likely that each bound to different antigens involved in different cell functions. Competition-binding assays were carried out to test this. Binding of radioiodinated JG9 or JG22 antibody was not reduced by competition with any of the other 12 antibodies. However, JG22, as either whole antibody or as monovalent Fab fragments, could inhibit the binding of JG9. Reciprocally, JG9 inhibited the binding of JG22. This surprising result suggests that JG9 and JG22 bind overlapping or even identical determinants or that they bind to sites so near each other on the cell surface that there is steric hindrance. The interesting experiment of adding the 2 antibodies in combination to living cultures is presently underway.

CHARACTERIZATION OF THE ANTIGEN BOUND BY JG9 AND JG22

• Experiments were undertaken to identify the antigen(s) bound by JG9 and 22. One approach used was to form a stable antibody-antigen complex at 4°C on living cells, extract the complex with detergents, and pass the extract over an A0.5 column with a molecular-weight cutoff at about 200,000. Free antibody was retarded by the column, whereas the antibody-antigen complex eluted in the void volume.

Another approach was to label metabolically muscle cell proteins with [^{35}S]methionine, prepare NP-40 extracts, and pass them over affinity columns of JG9, JG22, MOPC-21, or other monoclonal antibodies coupled to Sepharose beads. Bound molecules were eluted with low-pH buffer. SDS-polyacrylamide gel electrophoresis analysis of material passed twice over either a JG9 or JG22 column showed enrichment for a band of about 138,000 daltons and also for actin.

This 138,000-dalton band can also be detected without radiolabeling. Membrane pellets of embryonic muscle were extracted with NP-40, passed twice over a JG22 column, and the low-pH eluate was analyzed by Coomassie blue staining of SDS-polyacrylamide gels. Again, the 138,000-dalton band and actin were enriched. In all experiments using antibody affinity columns, the 138,000-dalton band was not enriched in eluates from MOPC-21 columns or columns of other monoclonal antibodies besides JG22 and JG9.

These biochemical studies show that a band of about 138,000 daltons is specifically bound by both JG9 and JG22 and that it is present in both cultured muscle and muscle in the developing embryo.

CONCLUSIONS

• Of the 14 surface-directed monoclonal antibodies examined, 12 did not disturb myogenic development when cells were cultured in the continual presence of the antibodies. We conclude that antibody binding per se need not lead to major changes in cell behavior. Two antibodies were found that do have dramatic effects on cell shape. The best characterized of these, JG22, appears to bind to a previously undescribed 138,000-dalton membrane protein. The other antibody, JG9, may also bind to this protein, but more evidence is needed to establish this point firmly. The activity of these antibodies is reversible in that normal cell shape is restored when the antibodies are withdrawn.

The major question raised by this study is, What is the mechanism of action of antibodies JG9 and JG22. Muscle cells in culture do not simply bind to the plastic dishes but have complex requirements for attachment. Collagen, fibronectin, and glycosaminoglycans have been clearly implicated as being involved in the adhesion of muscle cells to tissue culture dishes (Hauschka and Konigsberg 1966; Chiquet et al. 1979; Schubert and LaCorbier 1980). Perhaps the antibodies block the interaction of the 138,000-dalton proteins with these components. Alternatively, given the importance of the cytoskeleton in maintaining cell shape, the antibodies may disturb cytoskeletal structure. This model would imply that the 138,000-dalton antigen is a transmembrane link to the cytoskeleton.

Quite apart from the mechanism by which these antibodies change cell shape, their effects must be remembered when searching for antibodies that block more complex functions, such as synapse formation. Antibodies could block synaptogenesis indirectly by affecting the adhesive properties or shape of the muscle cell.

ACKNOWLEDGMENTS

• This study was supported by Public Health Service grant NS12867 and by a grant from the Muscular Dystrophy Association. D.G. was the recipient of a Research Career Development Award.

REFERENCES

Chiquet, M.E.E., C. Puri, and D.C. Turner. 1979. Fibronectin mediates attachment of chicken myoblasts to a gelatin-coated substrate. *J. Biol. Chem.* **254**:5475.

Frazier, W.B. and L. Glaser. 1979. Surface components and cell recognition. *Annu. Rev. Biochem.* **48**:491.

Galfre, G., C. Howe, C. Milstein, G.W. Butcher, and J.C. Howard. 1977. Antibodies to major histocompatibility antigens produced by hybrid cell lines. *Nature* **266**:550.

Gottlieb, D.I. and L. Glaser. 1980. Cellular recognition during neural development. *Annu. Rev. Neurosci.* **3**:303.

Hauschka, S.D. and I.R. Konigsberg. 1966. The influence of collagen on the development of muscle clones. *Proc. Natl. Acad. Sci.* **55**:119.

Schlessinger, J.E., E.L. Elson, W. Webb, I. Yahara, U. Rutishauser, and G.M. Edelman. 1977. Receptor diffusion on cell surfaces modulated by locally bound concanavalin A. *Proc. Natl. Acad. Sci.* **74**:1110.

Schubert, D. and M. LaCorbiere. 1980. A role of secreted glycosaminoglycans in cell-substratum adhesion. *J. Biol. Chem.* **255**:11,564.

Index

Acetylcholine (ACh)
  synaptic vesicle marker, 153–156
  secretion of, 182
  release of, 248
Acetylcholine receptor (AChR), 8,
    142, 193–194, 247–255,
    259
  localization, 266–267
Acetylcholinesterase, at synapse,
    247–255
ACh. *See* Acetylcholine
AChR. *See* Acetylcholine receptor
Acinar cells, 213–214
Action potential,
  in rat CNS lines, 39–40
  in hybrid cells, 244
Adenylatecyclase activation, 147,
    150
Adrenal chromaffin cell staining, 65,
    157, 176
Adrenal medulla, 176–177, 214
α-Bungaratoxin, 157
  and ACh, 198–201, 249, 261, 266
Amacrine cells, peptide staining, 203
Ambystoma tigrinum, 223
Amine production, uptake, and
    decarboxylation (APUD),
    209

Amines, with peptides in neurons,
    109
Aminopterin, 5, 260
Ammonium sulfate precipitation,
    144, 260
Androctonus a. Hecto, 30
APUD. *See* Amine production,
    uptake, and decarboxylation
Astrocytes, 17, 18, 21, 24
  antibody to GFAP-positive, 16,
    44–48
  anti–49K staining in, 24
  of corpus callosum, 128
  cytoplasmic markers, 17–19
  phosphocellulose and, 136
  in sciatic nerve, 22
  staining of intermediate filaments,
    128, 165
  staining in optic nerve, 63, 128
  vimentin in, 122

Basal lamina
  antigens and synapse organization,
    1, 259, 269
  neuromuscular synapse in, 1, 248,
    269
β_2-microglobulin, histocompatability
    antigens, 69